Wayfinding for Health Care

Best Practices for Today's Facilities

RANDY COOPER

HEALTH FORUM, INC.
An American Hospital Association Company
Chicago

This publication is designed to provide accurate and authoritative information in regard to the subject matter covered. It is sold with the understanding that neither the author nor the publisher is engaged in rendering legal, accounting, or other professional services. If legal advice or other expert assistance is required, the services of a competent professional should be sought.

The views expressed in this publication are strictly those of the author and do not represent the official positions of the American Hospital Association.

AHA and American Hospital Association are service marks of the American Hospital Association used under license by Health Forum, Inc.

Copyright ©2010 by Health Forum, Inc., an American Hospital Association company. All rights reserved. No part of this publication may be reproduced, stored in a retrieval system, or transmitted, in any form or by any means—electronic, mechanical, photocopying, recording, or otherwise—without the prior written permission of the publisher.

Printed in the United States of America

Cover design by Cheri Kusek

ISBN: 978-1-55648-369-1

Item Number: 055379

Project Management: Joyce Dunne
Editorial Assistance: Barbara Novosel
Photograph Editing: Jessica Lazar
Design and Typesetting: Fine Print, Ltd.
Production Management: Martin Weitzel
Acquisitions and Development: Richard Hill

Library of Congress Cataloging-in-Publication Data
Cooper, Randy.
   Wayfinding for health care : best practices for today's facilities / Randy Cooper.
      p. ; cm.
   Includes bibliographical references and index.
   ISBN 978-1-55648-369-1 (alk. paper)
   1. Health facilities—Design and construction. 2. Signs and signboards. I. Title.
   [DNLM: 1. Hospital Design and Construction. 2. Architectural Accessibility. 3. Location Directories and Signs. 4. Organizational Case Studies. WX 140 C778w 2010]
   RA967.C615 2010
   725'.51—dc22
                                                                          2009050446

Discounts on bulk quantities of books published by Health Forum, Inc., are available to professional associations, special marketers, educators, trainers, and others. For details and discount information, contact Health Forum, Inc., 155 North Wacker Drive, Chicago, IL 60606 (Phone: 1-800-242-2626).

*I am humbled at the thought of all those to whom
I need to dedicate this book.*

It is dedicated first to my lord and savior, Jesus Christ, for a lifetime of blessings with a drop of God-given talent.

I also want to dedicate it to my wife, Vickie, who is my soul mate, best friend, supporter, partner, and sometime critic.

I owe a great debt to all of those who have contributed to this project. They are a wonderful group of colleagues, writers, and editors who have made a graphics guy into a wordsmith.

Thanks to all the designers, "sign guys," and health care leaders who have come before me and worked alongside me. Many of these individuals pioneered the industry, and they set the bar very high. I have striven to learn from every employer, every employee, every business venture, and every client. I also want to thank in advance those who will build upon this work, thereby enriching patient care environments.

And last, but certainly not least, I dedicate this book to the staff of the American Hospital Association, who asked me to put this work together. I appreciate their support of me and of this project.

Contents

List of Figures

Chapter 8 also includes numerous photographs illustrating each of the case examples. However, these have been presented as collages with captions but without the formality of figure numbers or titles.

About the Author

Randy Cooper is an award-winning designer, a frequent speaker at health care events, and the owner and president of Cooper Sign & Graphics (CS&G) in Atlanta.

In the mid-1970s, when architectural firms were becoming "multidisciplined," a large firm in Ohio hired Mr. Cooper fresh out of Columbus College of Art and Design. His role was to become a project manager for the small graphics group that developed image packages, signage, and marketing aids for a wide range of business parks and retail and health care facilities. From the beginning, he recognized the need for collaborative efforts to make projects successful, which often meant interfacing with architects; engineers; and landscaping, planning, and business resources.

In 1979, Mr. Cooper accepted a position as vice president with a large Missouri sign company to design and develop new "architectural" products. This experience resulted in national and regional retail accounts serving the hospitality and health care fields.

Based on this experience, he accepted a job opportunity with ASI Sign Systems, the world's largest franchisee network of architectural signage. After serving initially in national franchisee training, Mr. Cooper became co-owner of a franchise in Sacramento, California.

In 1986, he sold his interest in that business and relocated to Atlanta to open a graphic design studio and to broker signage focusing on health care. Over the years, CS&G (as it came to be known) has evolved into a nationally recognized leader in design and fabrication of wayfinding and signage. Honors and recognition have included ranking the last three years as one of the top five sign companies nationally for the health care industry; sole endorsement by AHA Solutions, a division of the American Hospital Association; and two design awards for best new signage product for health care. Mr. Cooper has published eight articles in magazines with national circulations.

Foreword

My life in the sign industry began in the early 1960s with the formation of Custom Sign Company with my identical twin brother, Stanley. In 1968, we changed the company's name to Architectural Signing Inc. and then, in 1977, formed ASI Sign Systems. Although we are no longer involved with ASI, it is today the largest vendor of architectural sign solutions in the United States.

In my forty-five-plus years in this industry, obviously, I have seen many changes. In the early days, signage was usually an afterthought of the project architect, inserted into a section of the specifications called "Identifying Devices." Typically these were engraved signs. As the terms *signage, wayfinding,* and *environmental graphic design* were not yet in use in the architectural world, very little thought was given to creating a cohesive sign system, especially in hospital architecture.

The signage industry really started to change in the early 1970s with the formation of the Society of Environmental Graphic Design (SEGD), the professional organization for our industry. I first met Randy Cooper in the early 1980s when he was a co-owner of the ASI Sign Systems franchise in Sacramento, California. We worked together on many health care projects during this period and again during the 1990s, after he had formed his own company. It was during this time that the Americans with Disabilities Act became law, leading to considerable change in the sign industry.

In 1988, the annual SEGD Conference focused on the importance of wayfinding in the design of buildings, with an emphasis on health care facilities. In 1992, the book *Wayfinding: People, Signs, and Architecture,* by Paul Arthur and Romedi Passini, was published. While the authors credit Kevin Lynch with first using the word *wayfinding* in his 1960 book, *The Image of the City,* they note that it had no immediate influence on signage and graphics. But their book certainly did.

Recent research, wrote Arthur and Passini, "demonstrated that in a [hospital] facility of some 800 beds, no less than 8,000 hours of professional time are lost in redirecting patients and visitors to their destinations." Furthermore, "This is exclusive of the time that the professionals themselves lose in trying to find their way about, particularly when they are new on the job. . . . Nor does it refer to the hidden costs that result from delayed professional interventions, which may critically affect patients. Now, as every administrator knows, 8,000 hours of professional time represents at least 4 person-years—with all that implies."

Throughout the years, I have remained in close contact with Randy and have watched his growth as an expert in health care wayfinding and signage. From his early years as a graphic designer in architectural firms to holding key positions with both large commercial and architectural sign firms, his unique experience allows him a designer's perspective with the pragmatic approach of a seasoned sign fabricator. I take great pride in being asked to write the foreword for what is, in my opinion, the best and most complete book of its type ever written.

Indeed, there is nothing else like it. Other books on wayfinding are oriented to the design community—and none focuses on health care facilities, which clearly are a special case. Complex medical terminology, an almost haphazard pattern of expansion, organizational silos, and the stress levels of most patients and visitors make hospitals particularly difficult to navigate. Add to that situation today's heightened competitiveness and the shift from inpatient to ambulatory care, and organizations feel fresh urgency to differentiate themselves, expand their market share, build new facilities, and create a new image. All of this effort plays a part in an effective wayfinding program, which encompasses a lot more than just signs.

Wayfinding for Health Care will be helpful to graphic designers and architects with health care clients. But its primary purpose is to help health care executives and key management staff find their way to the *right wayfinding system for their own facilities*. With the information in this book, readers will gain the knowledge and confidence they need to:

- Oversee the development or revision of a program to suit the current and future needs of a hospital or other health care organization
- Make the case for funding and implementing such a program to a board and/or executive committee
- Identify, prioritize, and document wayfinding needs
- Evaluate different program options
- Hire and deal intelligently with wayfinding designers and sign vendors
- Improve and measure program performance

Randy Cooper, as might be expected, has used graphics to tremendous effect in this book, allowing readers to immediately *see* examples of what he is describing. Case examples illustrate how other health care organizations have put wayfinding principles into practice—and the results they have achieved.

Readers may or may not have the opportunity to work with Randy's team in the future. But once they have read this book, they will always have the benefit of his experience.

Hanley Bloom
Vice President, Sales
Neiman and Company
Van Nuys, California

Preface

Wayfinding is a user experience, a process, a plan, and a system.

Wayfinding as a user experience. Wayfinding historically refers to the user experience of orientation and choosing a path, self-navigating through the user's surroundings from point to point along a predetermined route. The self-navigation process relies on personal history, architectural elements, signage, maps, and other communicative tools—clues inherent in the built and natural environments' special grammar.

Wayfinding as a process. Wayfinding as a process generates a design solution, providing aids to the intuitive and deductive navigational process. These aids become clues to enhance the built and natural space; they can be as basic as dead reckoning, or they can integrate complex technology, such as touch screen computers and global positioning system devices. Tools often include maps/user guides, audible communication/written directions, tactile elements, consistent simplistic terminology, and environmental graphics.

Wayfinding as a plan. An effective wayfinding plan recognizes the human factor in the equation, bringing communications to their lowest common denominator, including provisions for users unfamiliar with their environment; under stress; and often with special needs, such as limited English proficiency or poor eyesight.

Wayfinding as a system. Implementing a wayfinding program takes careful orchestration, preplanning, and commitment, but the results are worth the effort.

HOW TO READ THIS BOOK

Several very good books have been written on wayfinding, and most have a chapter or a section on health care. This book is dedicated exclusively to wayfinding at health care facilities, big and small.

As a tool, the book is to be digested in layers, depending on how deeply you, the reader, choose to get involved. It is intended to be not so much a comprehensive do-it-yourself manual as a reference guide for health care executives, managers, and designers to stimulate thought and provide ideas that will get wayfinding projects on track quickly. In addition, it is strongly recommended as a handbook for members of wayfinding committees.

I suggest the book be read once through for the reader to become acquainted with the topic and various dimensions of wayfinding. This will provide a starting point for pursuing a particular area of interest. Chapters 1 through 3 deal with recognizing the problems and obtaining measurable data that will target needs and build understanding as to what wayfinding is, and is not. With that foundation, the reader will be ready to select a project team and direction to move forward to planning and designing (chapter 4) and implementing a wayfinding program (chapter 5) as appropriate.

Chapter 6 discusses codes and standards; it is not meant to be comprehensive but to emphasize the significance of codes and standards in wayfinding. This is an area in which you must be proactive, and this chapter allows you to learn from my experiences. Chapter 7 discusses wayfinding in health care facilities other than hospitals.

Many health care executives feel their facilities fall into one of two extremes in regard to wayfinding:

1. Our facility is unique and so screwed up that fixing it is overwhelming and impractical.
2. All facilities have these problems, and they are not worth tackling.

The lesson to be learned from the case examples in chapter 8 is that, while each facility is unique in its problems, these problems fit common, broad categories, and they are fixable. Our sample facilities show how others have tackled their wayfinding problems and been successful, regardless of their situation.

To facilitate your wayfinding pursuits further, the book includes a glossary of various wayfinding terms found in the book. You may not be familiar with every term, but you might be exposed to one or more of them during your wayfinding discussions.

I am thankful to the following individuals for assisting me in preparing this book for publication: Lauren Philips, editing; Jay Tokar, illustrations; and Dave Stewart, text contributor.

Wayfinding is part art, part science, and somewhat subjective. No matter whether you have been involved in wayfinding for a day or for years, this book is a tool that will help you with the journey. Good luck, and let me know your results and questions.

Randy Cooper
rcooper@wayfindingforhealthcare.com

Wayfinding
for Health Care

Wayfinding in Hospitals: A Special Challenge

After nine long months, Mr. Stringer's wife is finally in labor. Following his carefully planned route to the labor and delivery entrance of the community hospital, he finds that, because it is "after hours," he needs to redirect himself to the emergency department (ED). Once there, he parks in the ED short-term parking lot, escorts his wife inside, dashes back out to move his car to the main parking lot on the other side of the building, parks, and goes in the main entrance.

Since the ED is on the lower level, he needs to find the elevators. However, the elevators in the first bank he finds only travel up into the tower and not down to the lower level. The next bank is for staff use only. On his third try he finds the right one. Arriving back at the ED, he finds that his wife has already been taken up to the birthing suite in the labor and delivery department. He remembers visiting that area on the preregistration tour but doesn't remember where exactly it is in

Design is in everything we make, but it's also between those things. It's a mix of craft, science, storytelling, propaganda, and philosophy. Eric Adigard

the hospital. He never saw the ED on the tour, so he doesn't even know where he is in relation to the birthing suite. Thankfully, the ED staff are happy to tell him to take the second bank of elevators up to room 302 in the east wing. The ED, of course, is in the west wing. All he has to do is find the bridge between the two wings. What floor was that on?

On his way to the east wing he remembers he was supposed to call his mother-in-law, but in his rush, he has forgotten his cell phone at home. Surely the hospital still has pay phones. But where? Having searched for what seems an eternity to find a telephone; find change for the phone; get back to the phone; and then, mission accomplished, make his way to his wife's room, he finds that he is too late for the birth—something he will be hearing about even after the child has grown up and has children of her own.

Now that his wife and newborn daughter are resting, he at least has time to get a badly needed cup of coffee. Now where was that cafeteria . . . ?

◄ ►

The birth of a child is one of the few happy reasons people go to the hospital, and even then, excitement and anxiety can fog navigation skills. Almost all the rest of the reasons—including visiting someone else—involve worry at best, panic at worst, and often liberal doses of depression or guilt to heighten the stress. If ever a place needs clear, uncomplicated wayfinding, it is the hospital.

Unfortunately, few places are as confusing as a hospital. Older and more established hospitals and medical centers, by their very nature, are often put together like a poorly designed puzzle. They have been expanded, added on to, and reorganized without any thought to the original wayfinding intent. Even the venerable community hospital where "all the kids were born" will have made many bewildering changes by the time the parents bring their oldest child back for his first stitches. Of course, fewer adult Americans live in their childhood hometown these days, and that means many people first become familiar with the local hospital when they arrive filled with panic and in crisis mode.

WHAT MAKES HOSPITALS SO HARD TO NAVIGATE?

It is a fallacy to think that only the largest, oft-expanded urban or academic hospitals are difficult to navigate. We tend to think of smaller hospitals as being inherently more user friendly, but this thinking is not necessarily correct. Any size hospital can be a nightmare to navigate for anyone, from an anxiety-filled, panicky family member of a patient to a seasoned physician trying to find a department she never visits.

Conversely, any hospital can be made a breeze to navigate. Furthermore, this attention to easy wayfinding goes a long way toward making the hospital appear inviting and professional, if not warm, for all its visitors. To reach this goal, leaders must have the right attitude and enlist the expertise needed to make decisions about and deal with a few pesky peculiarities. The following sections illustrate the types of problems that exacerbate wayfinding shortcomings in many hospitals.

Terminology

Otolaryngology? PACU? As if the language of medicine isn't opaque enough to laypeople, it is also notoriously inconsistent, even within a single facility. Is the department called Imaging, Radiology, or X-ray? It depends. The sign that says X-ray may be old, or the person providing directions may prefer to call it Radiology. While *imaging* is a perfectly ordinary word to a health care professional, it is meaningless to many laypeople—the very people visiting to use the service. The inevitable changes of terminology can endlessly confuse a person who does not regularly visit the hospital. Sending someone to Community Services can stop a visitor cold if the department previously was called Public Relations.

Procedure versus Destination

Visitors to the facility may confuse the procedure they are scheduled to undergo with the department where they are to undergo it. This problem is related to terminology as well. If staff do not specify the name of the department(s) the patient must visit for the procedure, but rather just tell him that he is having a stress test performed, he may wander around the facility looking for the Stress Test Department when his actual destinations are, first, Outpatient Registration and then, Cardiology. Cleary, multiple destinations may exacerbate the wayfinding problem.

Dynamic Nature of Medicine

Just since lunch, entire specialties have emerged based on new technology to which patients are completely oblivious. New procedures, like fluorescence-assisted resection and exploration (FLARE), performed using a portable imaging system with no moving parts that makes no contact with the patient, are entirely alien to laypeople. When a patient is scheduled for this procedure, she may have no idea where to go to receive it. Even if she knows what FLARE is, she may not know what department in the hospital would house the machine.

Constant Expansion

The expansion of hospitals can lead to some baffling questions for patients. Health care facilities no longer have a single-building main entrance; rather, multiple "main entrances" serve new wings and other unconnected buildings across a large complex. Hospitals have grown into large systems that include far-flung campuses and isolated outposts across an entire town. Is the Women's Health Center a part of the main hospital or in a medical complex across town?

The confusion does not end when the patient arrives at the correct building. Naturally, a person assumes that wherever he enters a building is the first floor, the main level. But in today's hospitals, this is often not true. The situation is further complicated by the fact that the elevators serving the parking deck or garage may not align with those of the facility.

Good Move! When lack of a comprehensive master plan forced one burgeoning facility to locate a parking area a great distance from the main entrance, it made the best of a bad situation by placing inviting rest stations at even intervals, complete with benches, direct phones to assistance, clearly marked maps, and even defibrillators.

Someone looking for the hospital lobby parks on level 1 of the garage and may have to take an elevator up three floors to get the first floor of the hospital; if the lobby is on the second floor, another confusing selection of elevator buttons may present itself.

Constant Restructuring

Due to hospital restructuring brought about by change and growth, facility signage is often not updated frequently to reflect each change and help people find their way. Consider this example. A hospital adds a new labor and delivery suite but unintentionally confuses patients by moving the entire labor and delivery unit from the fourth floor to the fifth floor

and to a different side of the building. At the same time, the orthopedics department has been split in two to accommodate a new hand treatment–specific unit. In addition, this barrier means that some patients can no longer visit the physical therapy area in the same building. Getting lost on the way to physical therapy is an additional burden for those who are disabled, even temporarily.

Differences in Design, Scale, and Orientation

Sometimes staff use distinctions while giving directions that mean nothing to the patient or visitor. Once inside a hospital, people who do not work there have great difficulty determining if they are, for example, in the north tower or in the new (as opposed to the newly refurbished) section. To the public, hospitals tend to add wings, suites, units, floors—not to mention whole buildings with or without connecting hallways or bridges—in a seemingly random fashion over time. As a result, a visitor can abruptly turn a corner into what appears to be a completely different architectural environment. Inconsistent or overlapping room numbering can complicate the situation further.

Indistinguishable Decor

On the opposite end of the architectural environment spectrum, the hospital may feature endless identical corridors—often a testament to thrifty paint buying by maintenance—which can make visitors feel they are trapped in a tan maze. An individual has even more difficulty getting oriented within a labyrinth where every department looks the same. What decision does a visitor make when choosing between two hallways that look exactly the same?

Unexplained Protocols

Patients can sometimes find themselves in the wrong location because they received poor or inadequate information about the steps related to their appointment. Imagine sitting in the waiting room for 25 minutes, only to hear the following: "Did you check in first with Radiology?" "Did you pick up your paperwork already?" "Does the lab know you're here?" "You'll have to go to After Hours Care—you know, in the new wing."

Elevators with Restricted Access

Limiting access to certain areas to meet infection control, confidentiality, security, and other needs often means that hospital elevators do not stop on all floors, or, if they do, visitors run into barriers that require them to go back to the start and try again. They may have to transfer elevators, even elevator banks, to get to their destination. Poorly marking elevators as "Restricted Access" or not offering directions on the proper public elevator to use lead to a variety of problems.

Around-the-Clock versus Limited-Access Entrances

As poor Mr. Stringer found out in the story at the start of this chapter, directions given by staff or those available in hospital literature or online usually reference weekday hours, typically Monday through Friday from 9:00 AM to 5:00 PM. Because patients and visitors requiring services arrive at all hours, the proper information needs to be in their hands before their arrival.

Specialized Functions

The specialized functions within one department that seem intuitive to staff are often confusing to laypeople. Staff in one hospital, for example, could not understand why they kept coming across patients in the emergency department lobby with that deer-in-

the-headlights stare. A main cause of their confusion was that they were confronted with not one emergency care registration area but several: "scheduled" emergency care for those who had called ahead, urgent care, youth care, chest pain care, nurse-on-call care for after hours, and triage.

Crisis Mode

Patients cannot always know where to go in an emergency, especially if it involves a civic disaster. In the post-9/11 age, hospitals are expected to have comprehensive catastrophic care plans, which means an area designed as a lobby may have to be pressed into use as a triage area or some other function for which it was not designed.

Communications That Compete with Wayfinding Messages

Even after employing their best efforts to create a helpful wayfinding system, hospitals can still be a confusing place. The sheer number of communications that need to compete with wayfinding messages can become visual clutter. The more clutter in view, the less likely patients will notice the information they need. Some examples of visual clutter include these common signs:

- How patients are billed (with explanatory text)
- Restricted area
- How to get help
- The next blood drive is . . .
- To serve our patients better, we now offer . . . (introducing a new service)
- No smoking
- Please notify the technologist if you think you may be pregnant
- Please notify staff if your surgery is scheduled after 10 AM
- The lunch seminar topic today is . . .
- Out of service

Figure 1-1. Communications That Compete with Wayfinding Messages
Signage poorly done simply becomes visual clutter.

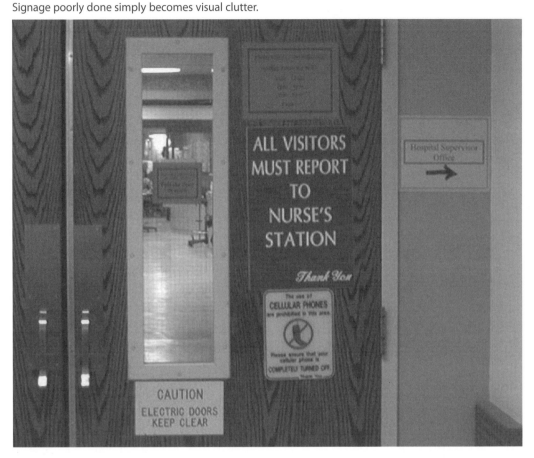

- Pardon our dust!
- Registration has been moved to 3A
- This area is being monitored by security
- Wet floor
- Patients' rights (with explanatory text)
- Flu shots now available

HOW DOES POOR WAYFINDING AFFECT HOSPITALS?

All of the problems introduced above lead to poor wayfinding, which in turn leaves a lasting emotional effect on patients and a lingering financial impact on hospitals. Hospitals are seen as places of confusion and anxiety for visitors, and as a result, revenue, referrals, and professional recruitment may suffer.

Simply put, when patients are lost, money is lost. Patients who are unsuccessful in their wayfinding arrive late for appointments. This delay causes downtime and disruption in schedules and staffing. Money is lost not only on idle staff but also on idle equipment whose expense cannot be recouped with nonbillable downtime. Physicians may have to reschedule other appointments and feel their time is being wasted.

Lost time can also come in the form of disruptions, which affect staff morale. Clinical and administrative staff lose time needed for their important jobs when they are constantly stopped and asked for directions.

Being lost undeniably leads to an increase in stress levels, which are already taxed by ill health or anxiety. The lost patient's level of satisfaction drops, and with it the organization's reputation. On average, twice as many people hear about a bad experience as hear about a good experience. Customer complaints take time and tact for staff to resolve, and those complaints are only the ones that staff hear about. Studies show that, for each complaint made, perhaps more than twenty other people are keeping their unhappiness to themselves—and to their friends, family members, coworkers, and fellow passengers on the bus.

Visibly and vocally disgruntled patients and visitors can cast a pall of gloom and tension over the facility. Add this feeling of communal dysfunction to the image of disorder that a visually cluttered facility projects, and a serious problem emerges, affecting patient and staff satisfaction and the bottom line. A facility that projects disorganization invites other forms of scrutiny.

Lost revenue, low patient satisfaction rates, and poor morale, however, all pale in comparison to the potential safety issues related to patients and visitors losing their way. Poor wayfinding can lead patients and visitors into restricted areas that can pose either a security problem or, worse, a hazard to their health and the health of others. Depending on the illness,

Figure 1-2. Poor Wayfinding as a Source of Confusion

As well as being hard to read, signs that fall into disrepair project a negative image.

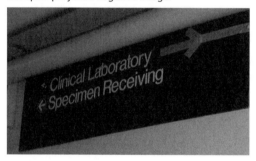

Figure 1-3. Poor Wayfinding as a Source of Anxiety

What is the impression formed by the architecture, design, and signage for this clinic space?

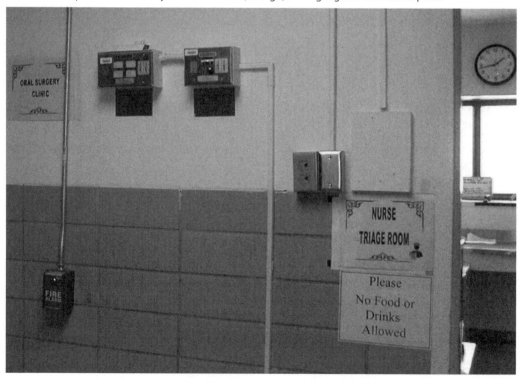

a patient can face a life-threatening situation if delayed, one that may also expose others to contamination or harm.

THE HUMAN FACTOR

A successful wayfinding program deals with more than giving directions and clearing visual clutter. The average person on the street may not be familiar with the word *wayfinding*, but it is both familiar and useful for architects, planners, and graphic designers as shorthand for all the ways people orient themselves in physical space and navigate from place to place.

The term was a gift from urban planner Kevin Lynch, who coined it in his book *The Image of the City* (MIT Press, 1960) to mean "a consistent use and organization of definite sensory cues from the external environment." The concept was later expanded by designer Paul Arthur and architect and environmental psychologist Romedi Passini in their book *Wayfinding: People, Signs, and Architecture* (McGraw-Hill, 1992) to encompass architecture, graphics, and verbal human interaction within the context of the built environment. The human element becomes more important when considering wayfinding in a hospital.

Whereas architects once designed for the "average"—a 5'3" woman weighing 135 pounds who read and spoke English, could read a map, and was right-handed—today they design for extremes, hoping to serve as wide a demo-

graphic as possible. As wildly various as people are, hospitals must find a common means of helping them get around highly complex

> **Don't Even Go There.** Sometimes signage can be more harmful than helpful. Overuse of restriction signs can project a negative impression. One facility wanted to remind visitors to lock their cars. In typical fashion, a committee sprang into action, the legal department got involved, and the sign that was posted said, "DO NOT LEAVE ANY VALUABLES IN CAR, KEEP CAR LOCKED AT ALL TIMES, SECURITY CAMERAS IN USE, HOSPITAL NOT RESPONSIBLE FOR LOSSES OR DAMAGE CAUSED TO VEHICLES. HAVE A NICE DAY." Technically, all information was correct and liability was limited, but it was not a very inviting message—in spite of the cheery afterthought.

facilities. To do so, they must take into account a number of human factors that can help or hinder the process. These factors are discussed in the following sections.

Physical Condition

Any hospital will be accessed by the occasional person who is, for example, deaf, who may have excellent powers of self-navigation but is at a distinct disadvantage if she must stop and ask for directions. A visitor's physical condition is especially important in hospitals, where people are often struggling with one or more handicaps such as a weakened heart, blurred vision, broken bones, failing muscles, and pain. At their best, many people—not all

> **Mixed Messages.** What could be more logical than to put that new wheelchair ramp at the back door of the hospital, where family members can drive right up to wait for discharged patients? The only problem is that the noisy loading dock and large, smelly Dumpster are at the same location, leaving those who cannot leave the hospital under their own power with a last (and lasting) impression of a real mess.

of them obese—cannot walk long distances or climb stairs.

Age

Many elderly people cannot see or hear well. Furthermore, often these problems are new to them and thus they are predisposed to confusion. Compounding their difficulty are suboptimal lighting conditions, high levels of ambient noise, and unfamiliar terminology. Elderly people tend to look down, take small steps, adjust to change slowly, and become disoriented quickly.

Reading Level

According to *The Informatics Review* (www .informatics-review.com), about 20 percent of the U.S. population is functionally illiterate; nearly half cannot read well enough to find a single piece of information in a short text, nor can they make low-level inferences based on what they read. Seventy-five percent of adult Americans with chronic health conditions scored in the lowest two literacy levels in a national literacy survey. Furthermore, even literate people are basically lazy readers, jumping to conclusions after just a few letters or words rather than taking in the whole word or sentence.

The Herd Instinct

The herd instinct is the tendency of people to follow a crowd, or even one very confident-looking person. Following the crowd typically means that people are not following the directions posted on signs.

Preconceptions

The laboratory is always in the basement, right? Americans are accustomed to using their experience to guide them, which can work well in big-box retail stores and shop-ping malls but trip them up when entering a new, reconfigured, or unfamiliar hospital, clinic, or doctor's office.

Emotional Responses

Many people feel light-headed, nauseous, or dizzy when they see needles, hear sirens, or smell disinfectant. Even seasoned medical staff may lose their nonchalance when blood is coming from a member of their own family. Fear can disrupt one's focus on instructions and impede direction following.

Previous Associations

It is hard to break old habits and unlearn previously acquired knowledge. People may become confused if the door on the south side of the hospital previously served as the general public entrance but now, with the expansion complete, is used for staff only. However, habits can work advantageously if all signs pointing toward the emergency department are red.

Respect for Authority

Another human factor that can lead to positive outcomes is a general respect for authority. People are usually willing to ask for directions when lost. In fact, most people have been trained since childhood to turn to a person in authority when lost. On the other hand, people who are asked for directions often feel the need to give them, even if they really are not sure of the answer or cannot explain the way well. In addition, many people have a hard time remembering exactly what they have been told. In the same way that many people are lazy readers, many are lazy listeners. A person may hear, "Take the stairs at the end of the first hall" and assume the way will become clearer at that point, so he promptly forgets whether the next move is a right or a left.

THE COGNITIVE MAPPING PROCESS

How does a wayfinding program go about solving all of the problems that hospitals face in getting their visitors and patients from here to there in a safe, pleasant, and timely fashion? Such movement typically involves a series of decision points. These points are often intersections in roads or halls, where the choices are right, left, up, down, and straight ahead, and where signs featuring words or symbols may suggest the right course. In between such points, however, we may need directional reinforcement to keep us moving on the right path.

The news is not all bad. Even without signs, maps, or hints, people usually have some sense of how to proceed, thanks to cognitive mapping, which may take place on a conscious or an unconscious level. In developing or enhancing a wayfinding program, an organization must keep in mind the common tools and techniques of cognitive mapping discussed in the sections that follow. A successful wayfinding program does not rewrite the book on how people operate. Instead, it capitalizes on some of these tools of cognitive mapping and helps people better employ their natural abilities.

Distance and Direction

This is the basic "Go about two miles and then turn east toward the center of town" approach, which relies on approximation, experience, and common sense. Studies show that people cannot grasp complex directions—they need instructions broken down into small bits of information. Think of this concept like a child completing a connect-the-dots puzzle: She draws from one dot to the next without seeing the entire picture until she reaches the end.

Landmarking and Placemaking

Some people orient better to specific physical landmarks, which can include unique symbols, colors, or other elements as well as structures and features of the landscape. "Turn left at the cafeteria, go up the blue stairs, and turn right at the fountain"—these symbols or design elements render a place as unique and special and allow it to stand out from the surrounding landscape.

Compass Orientation

"Turn north (right) at the brick building, then east (left) at the fountain" makes the most of what is, for some, a natural sense or ability. But not every one orients well to the compass, especially indoors, making it a risky faculty to rely on exclusively.

Dead Reckoning

To enter a shopping mall, dead reckoning tells us to drive around the exterior until we find a major anchor store, then park as close as we can. If you want people to move in a contrary fashion, subtlety will not achieve that goal. For example, knowing that the x-ray department is in the south wing is helpful only if the person can access the south wing from where he is and the way is not blocked by, say, an "authorized personnel only" area without any directions pointing to an alternate route.

Imagine a hospital with a north wing connected by a central corridor to a south wing. Visitors are frustrated to learn that they cannot travel from the fourth floor in the north wing to the fourth floor in the south wing using the central corridor. A drug rehabilitation unit is in the central corridor on the fourth floor. It is a restricted area that is locked down. The visitor's only choice is to get on an elevator and go to any of floors 1 through 3, travel through the central corridor, and then take an elevator back up to the fourth floor.

Dead reckoning makes people want to walk down that fourth floor central corridor. In this case, it is important to convey to visitors that they need to vertically circulate to get to the other side of the fourth floor.

Proximity, Direction, and Destination

The best directional system is often a hybrid of all these cognitive mapping methods. General information should be offered first ("Take this elevator to the third floor") followed by more specific information once a person reaches the correct floor ("Turn right for the laboratory") and positive reinforcement once she arrives ("This is the laboratory"). The challenge, of course, is to provide a wayfinding program that meets everyone at his or her own level. The program needs to take into account all of the human factors and all of the cognitive mapping methods people may use.

COMMON APPROACHES

In trying to meet everyone at his or her own level, many hospitals have used some combi-

nation of the elements described below. These approaches are the basics, but only the basics, of a successful wayfinding program. They pose problems of their own if used alone.

Color Stripes

Veterans Administration hospitals were among the first to paint multicolor lines on the floor to direct visitors to various areas. When it turned out that these lines were hard to update, some facilities went to color stripes on walls or even on ceiling tiles, which inevitably morphed into multicolored footprints along the floor or other icons placed on the wall. The more complex facilities became, the more colors they had to use and the harder it was (especially for the color blind) to distinguish among similar shades such as mauve/wine and green/teal.

Compass Orientation

Many facilities are deeply entrenched in a system that simply evolved. Perhaps the nursing unit on the third floor of the east wing became known as 3 East. With growth of the facility, however, come awkward designations like upper-3E or 6NE.

Figure 1-4. Signage for Compass Orientation
How do you know you have arrived at the correct wing without proper signage?

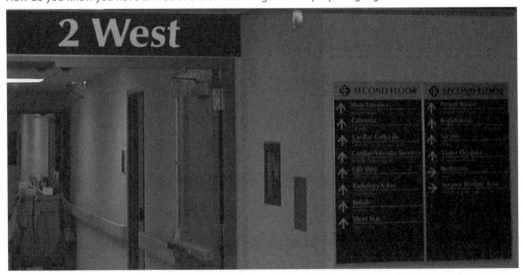

Quadrant/Wing/Area Systems

A more contemporary approach to wayfinding is to designate quadrants, wings, or major areas by alphabetical letters, numbers, or categorized names and icons. This system has considerable merit but requires both employee and visitor education and may not be able to stand alone without more traditional directional signage.

Construction Phrases

The use of construction-based phrases works well among staff and employees, but a term like "the tower" is not helpful to patients or visitors, while "the back of the hospital" or "the old part of the building" is positively off-putting.

Color Coding

While sharing many of the same problems as the old stripes-on-the-floors scheme, color coding can be useful as a method of reinforcement, especially when layered with other reinforcers. For example, the second floor of a parking structure might be designated as yellow and feature an icon of a canary or be designated Second/Yellow Floor in labeling and diagrams. Assigning colors that are closely related (such as purple and blue) to departments in the same general area is also a good approach. If someone has trouble distinguishing colors, he or she will at least be close to the destination.

Physical Addresses

Exterior elements can be named and mapped like roads, a system already familiar to almost everyone. This approach can be particularly helpful on large campuses, where destinations, stand-alone buildings, and parking areas can number in the hundreds. Even if two units within a large campus share one mailing address, they could each have unique address designations tied to a global positioning system (GPS) and online search engines as well as maps. Some facilities use a similar concept for the interior, literally naming hallways and even giving internal destinations separate addresses. "Go down Emergency Boulevard until you reach Clinic Road," say, "and then

Figure 1-5. Signage for Physical Addresses
Internal elements can be named and mapped like streets.

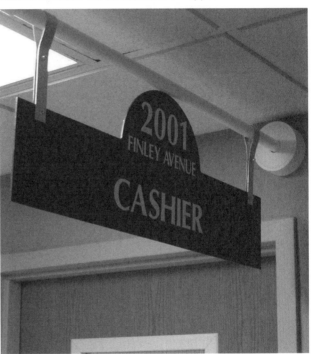

turn right until you get to Outpatient Registration, which is number 2402." This system can be effective, but only if the concept can be clearly and quickly conveyed to the average user.

Contained Positioning Systems

Contained positioning systems (CPS), similar to GPS but contained within a single building or complex, is on the wayfinding horizon. Handheld CPS devices are distributed to patients for use in navigating the facility. Wiring facilities to implement such a system will be relatively simple, but using it may present problems: Early tests have shown that people need help to program the proper destination, and confusion can arise when multiple destinations or a change in destination is involved. And the matter of keeping the handheld units from going home with the visitors is also a concern.

Avoiding the Las Vegas Syndrome

The idea is not to mix and match wayfinding solutions to suit individual elements of the facility but to craft a system that reflects the organization as a unified whole, that says "This is who we are." And while it may be tempting, and in many cases appropriate, to use many wayfinding approaches in combination, it is important to keep in mind that over-signing can be as much (if not more) of a trap as under-signing. The dangers are sensory overload, with multiple signs fighting for attention and blocking or overshadowing each other, and duplication, which can cancel out both messages. It is necessary to find the balance between no wayfinding system at all and visual clutter.

BUSTING THE COMMON WAYFINDING MYTHS

It is important to take wayfinding seriously. Many times people in hospital management make the mistake of thinking, "Our hospital has been here forever and all our visitors know where they are going" or "People will find their way, and if they don't, they'll ask for directions" or even "Once people are inside the building, our job is done." As this chapter has illustrated, these mind-sets lead to a loss of revenue; a loss of patient satisfaction; and

even threats to health, safety, and security for patients and staff alike.

Following are some common wayfinding myths often believed by hospital leaders that can be just as damaging as the mind-sets mentioned above:

- Planning for effective wayfinding is a luxury.
- Preparing an effective wayfinding plan is a small commitment.
- Only large, urban facilities need a wayfinding program.
- We can form a committee to "fix the problem" in-house.
- Bigger signs will take care of our wayfinding problem.
- More signs will take care of our wayfinding problem.
- Wayfinding is not an ongoing concern. It is a one-time fix.
- Wayfinding is only signage.

In fact, wayfinding is much more than putting up a few extra signs. It is a process that includes people, resources, and knowledge from departments hospital-wide. A wayfinding initiative needs preplanning. Once the plan is in motion, all of the players must work together to use all the necessary environmental materials and communicative tools. Finally, facility commitment is vital to both starting a wayfinding project and maintaining the plan so that it remains relevant and helpful in the future.

Preplanning

Preparing for an effective wayfinding plan is no small commitment. It is vital to include a preplanning stage in the process wherein a plan is devised, workable goals are established, and a final target goal is clearly defined. The Herculean effort in carrying out all the tasks in this step is not accomplished by one person alone. An in-house team, including a wayfinding committee, needs to be assembled (see chapter 3). This committee should consider inviting the facilities architect, interior designer, and possibly a landscape architect to participate in preplanning, as well as a design consultant, contractors, and subcontractors, who can provide valuable insights into the preplanning process.

Using Environmental Materials and Communicative Tools

Signs are important, but additional resources need to be available to create an effective wayfinding program. On the exterior of the hospital and across the campus, natural spaces and architectural features can and should be utilized. In the interior, furnishings, art, lighting, color, floor treatments, and other landmarks are all important elements of successful wayfinding.

In a wayfinding system, communicative tools include more than signage. The signage system should be comprehensive and consistent in its appearance and use of terminology. The signs should be integrated with printed maps and directions, electronic applications, and staff training. Wayfinding is good customer service.

Achieving Facility-Wide Commitment

Gaining complete, facility-wide commitment is the only way for a successful wayfinding initiative to be implemented and maintained. The wayfinding program needs to remain a priority because it will positively affect every department, staff member, and patient across the entire hospital. All facility resources need to be made available to the wayfinding team. Staff need to be trained to facilitate effective wayfinding in order for the program to have the highest impact both in the early days after

implementation and for years into the future as the hospital continues to grow and evolve.

CONCLUSION

Staff at many facilities mistakenly think their wayfinding system is simply too broken to fix—that they somehow have to live with the problem or put quick fixes in place on a case-by-case basis. Do not fall into the trap of believing that all the hospital needs is more— more and bigger signs, more maps, more volunteers to act as ambassadors escorting patients and visitors. While these efforts can help address a symptom, they do not address the illness.

Wayfinding problems arise from fundamental issues in communication and poorly evolved architecture. They are usually the result of a slow leak, not a deluge. Just as they have taken years to develop, wayfinding problems will take time to fix. But the rewards become evident quickly.

As the hospital looks to correct problems that relate to poor wayfinding in both the built and natural environments, solutions will involve several action items, and multiple tools will be needed. The remainder of this book is dedicated to taking some of the fear out of the improvement process and serving as a reference tool in the hospital's journey toward excellence in customer satisfaction and patient throughput.

Figure 1-6 summarizes the scope of hospital wayfinding. Each facility must choose its own methodology to address its wayfinding problems and determine how best to position itself based on its corporate needs, the uniqueness of the campus/facility, and the targeted ethnographic groups using the facility. Making an informed choice begins with an understanding of the tools of the trade.

Figure 1-6. The Scope of Wayfinding
Wayfinding is much more than signs. Because wayfinding is a facility-wide challenge, effective wayfinding integrates a facility-wide response.

Preplanning

- Involve Wayfinding Consultant
- Involve "In House" Team
- Involve Consultants and Contractors
- Involve Others as Appropriate
- Clearly Define Target
- Establish Workable Goals
- Devise Plan

Facility Commitment

- Maintain the Initiative as a Priority
- Make Data and Facility Resources Available
- Train Staff

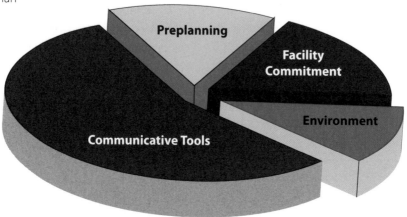

Communicative Tools

- Aimed at Target: Keep It Simple
- Comprehensive Signage System
- Consistency in Signage Appearance and Terminology
- Integrate Signage with:
  ▸ Printed Maps and Directions
  ▸ Electronic Applications
  ▸ Staff Training: Wayfinding Is Customer Service
- Information/Directions Given at Home and in Doctor's Offices

Environment

- Natural Spaces
- Architectural Features
- Interiors
- Furnishings
- Art
- Lighting
- Floor Treatments
- Other Placemaking Elements

Tools of the Trade

G lobal positioning system (GPS) devices, maps, user guides, interactive electronic kiosks, audible communication systems, written directions, Web sites, tactile elements, visual clues, a wide range of graphics—the list of the tools used in wayfinding programs can go on and on. All are designed to ease the navigational process, as one organization profiled in chapter 8 determined upon completing a cognitive mapping process (see figure 2-1). And while wayfinding is much more than just signage, signs are the tool that is most heavily relied on and, in many situations, the most poorly executed.

> When I am working on a problem, I never think about beauty. I think only of how to solve the problem. But when I have finished, if the solution is not beautiful, I know it is wrong.
>
> R. Buckminster Fuller

Figure 2-1. Sample Wayfinding Methodology
University Health Systems (UHS) of Eastern Carolina and East Carolina University (ECU),
Greenville, North Carolina, defined this wayfinding methodology from home to destination.
The methodology identifies a range of tools for easing the navigational process.

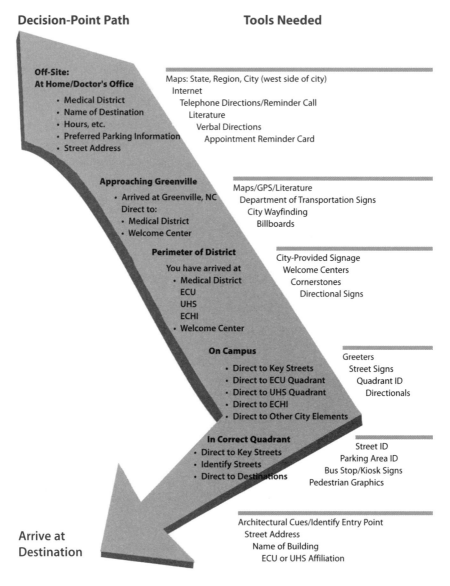

Decision-Point Path   **Tools Needed**

Off-Site:
At Home/Doctor's Office   Maps: State, Region, City (west side of city)
                                          Internet
- Medical District   Telephone Directions/Reminder Call
- Name of Destination   Literature
- Hours, etc.   Verbal Directions
- Preferred Parking Information   Appointment Reminder Card
- Street Address

Approaching Greenville   Maps/GPS/Literature
- Arrived at Greenville, NC   Department of Transportation Signs
Direct to: City Wayfinding
- Medical District   Billboards
- Welcome Center

Perimeter of District   City-Provided Signage
You have arrived at   Welcome Centers
- Medical District   Cornerstones
ECU   Directional Signs
UHS
ECHI
- Welcome Center

On Campus   Greeters
- Direct to Key Streets   Street Signs
- Direct to ECU Quadrant   Quadrant ID
- Direct to UHS Quadrant   Directionals
- Direct to ECHI
- Direct to Other City Elements

In Correct Quadrant   Street ID
- Direct to Key Streets   Parking Area ID
- Identify Streets   Bus Stop/Kiosk Signs
- Direct to Destinations   Pedestrian Graphics

Arrive at   Architectural Cues/Identify Entry Point
Destination   Street Address
                                                Name of Building
                                                 ECU or UHS Affiliation

Note: ECHI = East Carolina Heart Institute

SIGNAGE SYSTEMS

A consumer-friendly hospital does not simply have a lot of signs. It has a comprehensive signage *system*, in which each sign has a specific message to communicate and bears a strong familial resemblance to every other sign in the same facility.

These strong family resemblances designate the system's design and placement as part of a preplanned visual hierarchy. As with so much else in design, less is more. A sign should convey complete, accurate, and concise information as simply as possible. Each element should reflect its rank in importance.

> Always design a thing by considering it in its next larger context—a chair in a room, a room in a house, a house in an environment, an environment in a city plan.   Eliel Saarinen

Placement is a key factor in effective signage. It is not enough for a sign to be visible; it must draw the eye and compete successfully with artwork, safety notices, clocks, and a whole range of other important functional and aesthetic elements. Indeed, finding the right balance between function and aesthetics while avoiding visual clutter is a major challenge in hospital wayfinding.

The visual language that ties similar signs together is called a *lexicon*. When used properly, this language allows the reader of the sign to determine subliminally what a sign will tell her long before she is close enough to actually read it. A typical lexicon will constitute some or all of the elements shown in figures 2-2 and 2-3, sometimes combined into a hybrid sign type.

Figure 2-2. Basic Exterior Signage Lexicon Elements

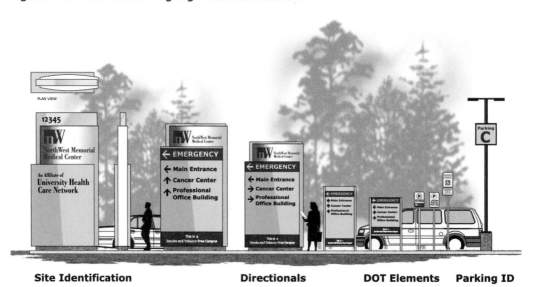

Site Identification   **Directionals**   **DOT Elements**   **Parking ID**

Vista Graphics

Building
Identification

Entry
Identification

Door Logos /
Door Bands

Figure 2-3. Supplemental Elements of the Lexicon

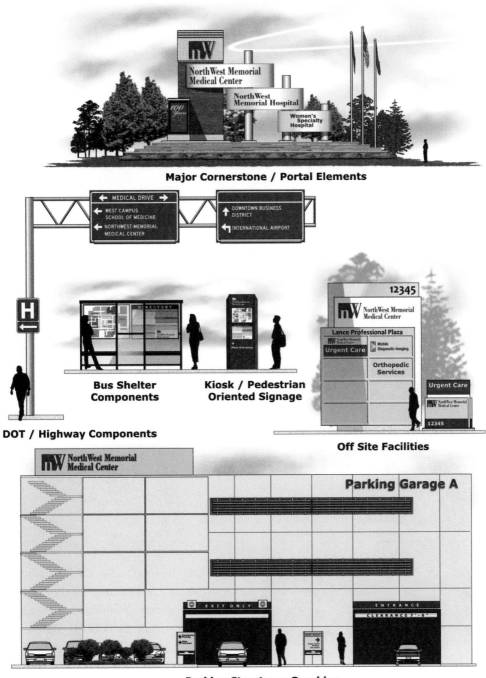

Major Cornerstone / Portal Elements

DOT / Highway Components

Bus Shelter Components

Kiosk / Pedestrian Oriented Signage

Off Site Facilities

Parking Structures Graphics

This chapter describes and shows examples of all the main signs and other tools that can be used in a wayfinding program. Imagine this chapter as a journey from off-campus to a desired location within a hospital. The examples first provide images of signs that are relatively distant from the hospital; then, progressively closer, those in proximity to the hospital; followed by signs in the hospital; and finally, signs directing visitors to individual departments and rooms.

EXTERIOR SIGNS

Figure 2-4. Trailblazer Sign

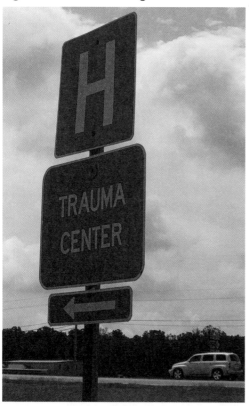

Trailblazer sign. This type of sign consists of the basic white H on a blue rectangular back-

ground, provided by or with the permission of the appropriate department of transportation (DOT) exclusively to direct traffic to the entrance of a 24-hour emergency facility. Some areas allow these signs to be personalized to distinguish facilities by name that are in close proximity to each other.

Figure 2-5. Vista/Campus Identification

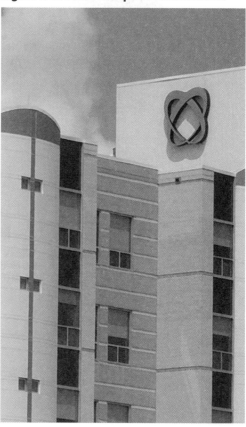

Vista/campus identification. Can the campus be seen from an expressway or a major highway? If so, then a strong statement of site or campus identification may be needed. Such a statement often takes the form of a large logo or the organization's initials high on a facility's wall so as to be visible from a good distance.

Figure 2-6. Major Cornerstones

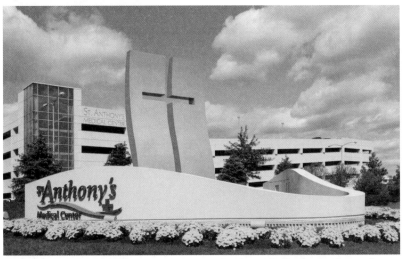

Major cornerstones. When campuses sprawl, with facilities dissimilar in architecture and function, they can quickly lose a sense of visual connectivity. A strong cornerstone element at the perimeters of the property can help define the presence of the campus. It also gives the first impression of the hospital brand long before a visitor enters a building.

Figure 2-7. Retail/Advertising

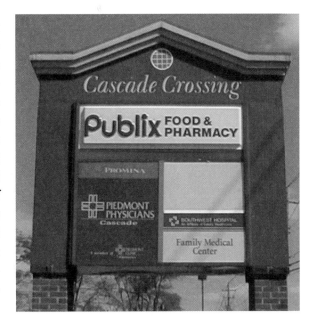

Retail/advertising. Remember to appropriately identify the off-site facilities connected to the hospital. It is important to continue to show the same attention to signs off-campus as is paid to those on-campus. Sometimes these signs need to share space with other retail signs. Architectural signing purists tend to downplay the advertising value of signage, both exterior and interior. The reality is that medically oriented retail facilities have to show a return on their investment to stay in business, and signage is a proven way to position themselves to that end.

Figure 2-8. Directories

Directories. Once on campus, the visitor finds exterior directories to be particularly helpful when they include maps along with a listing of offices.

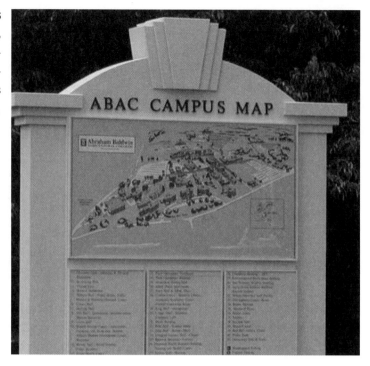

Figure 2-9. Vehicular/ Pedestrian Directional Sign: Primary

Figure 2-10. Vehicular/ Pedestrian Directional Sign: Secondary

Figure 2-11. Vehicular/ Pedestrian Directional Sign: Rudimentary

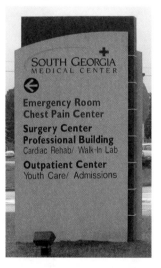

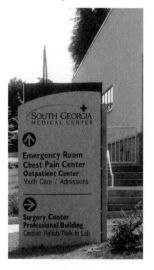

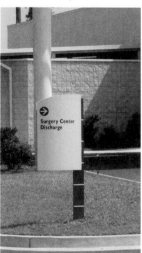

Vehicular/pedestrian directional signs. Scale and appearance vary in directional signage, but these signs serve the same purpose: to point visitors in the right direction. In figures 2-9, 2-10, and 2-11, visitors to South Georgia Medical Center, Valdosta, Georgia, are given directions to a variety of locations. The signs indicate the importance of the information they are conveying through color, letter size, and position on the sign. All three signs reinforce the logo and brand of the hospital before the visitor sets foot in the facility.

Directional signs do the pointing for you:

- Primary signs are used for the highest-priority messages and often for multiple destinations.
- Secondary signs are usually less complex or used for fewer messages; such signs are typically smaller but similar to primary directionals.
- Rudimentary signs are used for much more basic information; they often take a lower priority weight of all the vehicular directional signs.

Figure 2-12. Primary-Site Identification

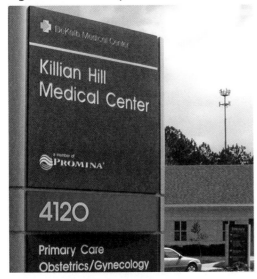

Primary-site identification. Each public building on- and off-campus needs to be singularly identified. It needs a unique name and an address, if one has been assigned. Street addresses for buildings are required by postal services and fire marshals. However, sometimes one address is assigned to an entire cam-

pus, and individual buildings on the campus do not have separate addresses. Now, with the use of GPS, addresses have an even wider wayfinding purpose.

These identification signs must signify the building as part of the whole. In figure 2-12, the sign clearly indicates that the Killian Hill Medical Center is part of the DeKalb Medical Center.

Figure 2-13. Tenant Identification

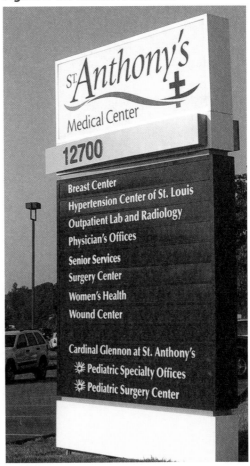

Tenant identification. Tenants are sometimes named on primary-site identification signs, but this practice can quickly lead to massive visual pollution and sensory overload.

Figure 2-14. Building Identification

Building identification. Unlike site identification signs, building identification signs are used for single buildings only. Whether freestanding or wall mounted, these signs identify the name of the building and, often, major tenants.

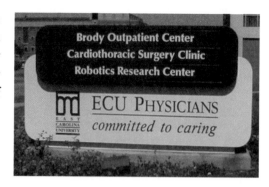

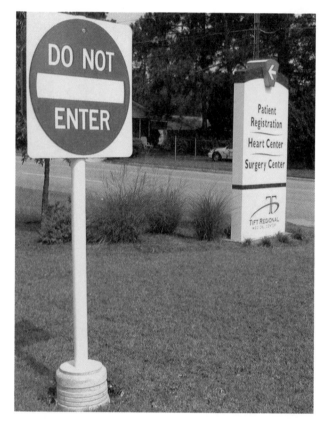

Figure 2-15. Department of Transportation Signage

Department of transportation signage. Driving around any hospital campus, both large and small, one views stop signs, street signs, speed limit signs, pedestrian crossing signs, and so forth, which are assigned or erected by the area DOT. Their shapes, colors, and mounting heights are specifically associated with their function. However, in recent years, an effort has been made to incorporate these utilitarian signs into the more graphically pleasing architectural sign system of facilities. It is important to remember, however, that the standard appearance of these particular visual elements should be maintained, both for legal reasons and to conform to people's expectations.

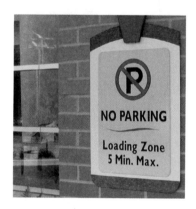

Figure 2-16. Regulatory/Policy Messages

Regulatory/policy messages. A significant aspect of effective wayfinding is to communicate a wide range of policy or regulatory messages that are either required by a governmental agency or dictated by hospital administration.

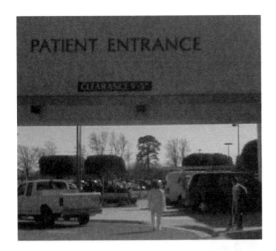

Figure 2-17. Clearance Limits

Clearance limits. Clearance limit signs, while not directly indicating direction, show visitors limitations to access and are also a part of the visual landscape.

Figure 2-18. Entrance Identification

Entrance identification. As a facility grows, its multiplying entrances add to user confusion. Do not count on architecture alone to define the correct entrance for the visitor; instead, use freestanding or wall-mounted/canopy signage to add clarity.

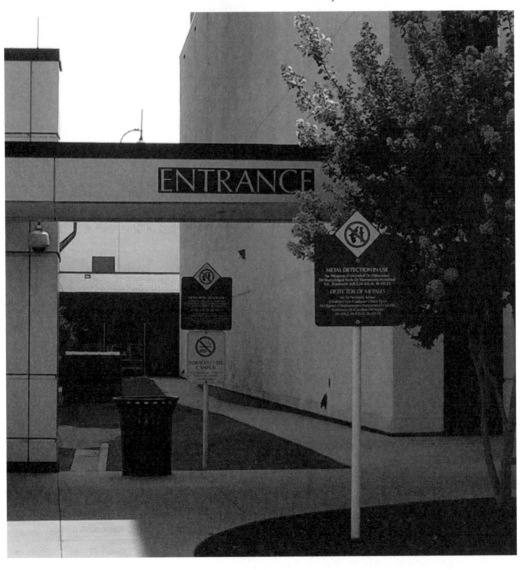

Figure 2-19. Entrance Door Graphics/Door Bands

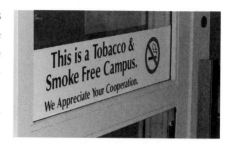

Entrance door graphics/door bands. Too often, signage systems do not include all essential information at the entryway, which should feature a facility logo; the designated name of the entrance; the hours of operation; and information on policies such as those dealing with smoking, attire requirements, and other restrictions.

INTERIOR SIGNS

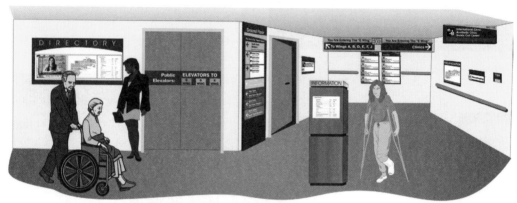

Figure 2-20. Typical Interior Lexicon

A typical interior lexicon reflects the familial resemblance and relative visual weighting of the various sign types. Each sign is designed to communicate specific types of information within the context of a unified systems approach.

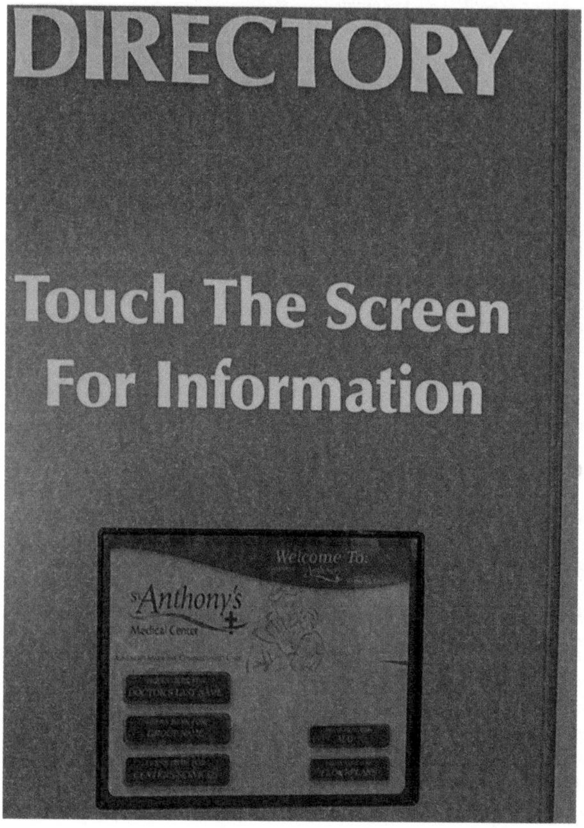

Figure 2-21. Building Directory

Building directory. Whether a simple changeable-letter unit or sophisticated touch screen technology, the directory must communicate who and what resides in the facility. Some facilities use maps and floor plans, but conventional wisdom is to not mix directory information—floor, suite number, wing, or quadrant—with arrows, which are better left for directional signs.

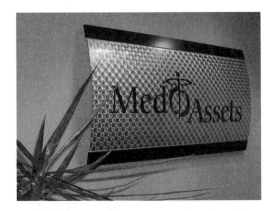

Figure 2-22. Lobby Graphics

Lobby graphics. Graphics may be used in a lobby to usher a visitor into an office atrium or out of an elevator to welcome him to a destination. The use of such graphics is a great opportunity to reinforce branding efforts.

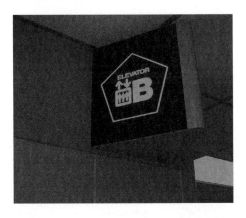

Figure 2-23. Elevator Designation

Elevator designation. Because hospitals grow in various phases, some elevators service only certain levels, while others are reserved for staff use or patient transport. Clearly labeling each elevator and indicating its destination is critical; it can help to thematically tie together all the landings that are serviced by a single elevator. Another common way to identify elevators is to provide door bands directly on the doors.

Figure 2-24. Secondary/Elevator-Specific Directories

Secondary/elevator-specific directories. When a person arrives at an elevator, she should expect to be met with a second, reinforcing directory. Elevator-specific directories are similar to whole-building directories but either are limited to or give priority to destinations accessible by way of that specific elevator.

Signage designed by HDR Architecture, Omaha, Nebraska, for East Carolina Heart Institute, Pitt County Memorial Hospital, Greenville, North Carolina.

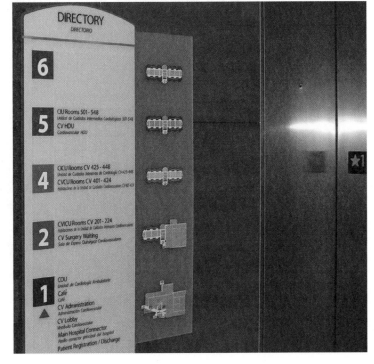

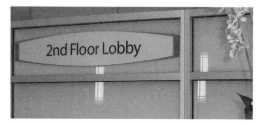

Figure 2-25. Level Identification

Level identification. With expansions, many hospitals end up with floor levels that do not align. A visitor may literally change levels simply by walking through a door or up a slight ramp, which is a cause for confusion. Furthermore, most people assume that wherever they enter a facility is the ground floor or level 1—again, with expansion or redesign, this assumption is not always correct. To help clarify these location discrepancies, display the floor level at key points such as in elevator lobbies and on directional signs.

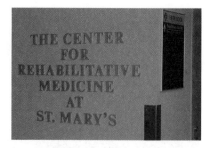

Figure 2-26. Area/Quadrant/ Wing Designation

Area/quadrant/wing designation. Different sections of a facility can be difficult for a first-time or infrequent visitor to distinguish (a tower is really only perceived as such from the outside), making it essential that areas, quadrants, and wings be clearly identified.

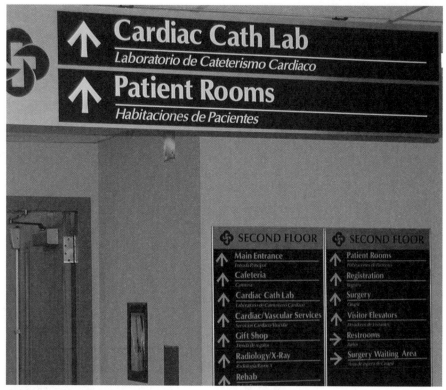

Figure 2-27. Directional Signs

Directional signs. Not to be confused with directories, which primarily move people vertically, these arrow signs (or "directionals") move people horizontally on just one level, like a trail of bread crumbs. They can be freestanding or mounted on the wall, ceiling, or transom, depending on the best line of sight. Directionals are needed at every decision point so that they work together as a chain. One missed link can cause serious problems in traffic flow.

Good Move! Think of directionals as a series of relays, passing the visitor from one decision point to the next, and possibly more detailed, decision point. Be cautioned that you should start listing multiple destinations on your directionals as an area nears; stick with one destination but gradually increase specificity. For example, initially, direct people toward Materials Management and then, as they get closer, split listings into director's office, loading dock, and so forth.

Figure 2-28. Placemaking/Environmental Graphics

Placemaking/environmental graphics. Graphic elements that may or may not include traditional signage elements can help make an area unique and memorable. Such elements might be a distinctive wall color ("Take this hall to the purple waiting room"), special lighting, or seating that stamps a space with its own theme.

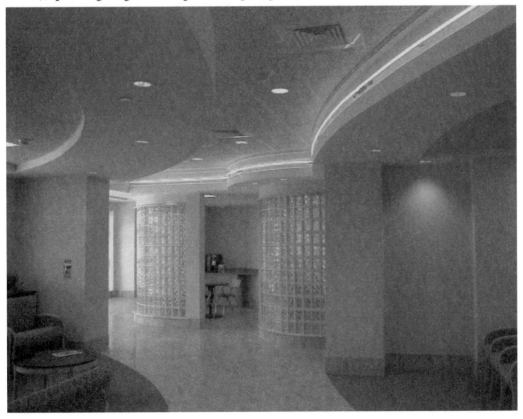

Figure 2-29. Department Identification

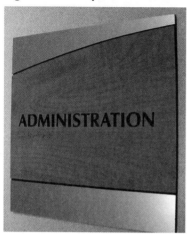

Department identification. Say a visitor knows where Administration is located. How does she know, however, when she has entered this area or department? Where is the "entrance"? Department identification signage marks this area definitively for the user.

Figure 2-30. Room Numbers

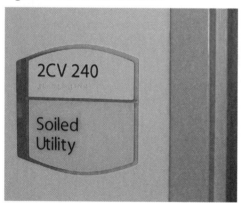

Signage designed by HDR Architecture, Omaha, Nebraska, for East Carolina Heart Institute, Pitt County Memorial Hospital, Greenville, North Carolina.

Room numbers. Numbers are needed by staff as well as patients and visitors to correctly identify a location. Most facilities do not have a comprehensive, facility-wide numbering system, but such a system can be a tremendous help in tracking or taking inventory of equipment and furniture and in submitting maintenance orders as well as in wayfinding. Number plaques can also incorporate bar codes for scanning purposes.

Figure 2-31. Room Identification: Primary

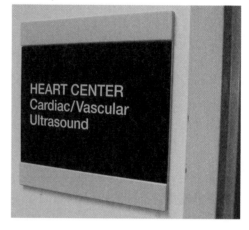

Figure 2-32. Room Identification: Secondary

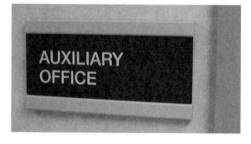

Room identification. When it comes to designating room function, terminology matters. If you choose a term like *storage*, then you must commit to assigning the location a two-hour fire rating. Primary and secondary room identification refer to areas that are more and less heavily used, respectively. Patient room signs typically are of a very specific type; they must accommodate patient care messages such as "patient prone to falls." Nursing services will need to be involved in deciding how these signs will be displayed.

Figure 2-33. Conference Meeting Rooms

Conference meeting rooms. In addition to providing room name or number, these signs should display information such as a meeting schedule or an in use/ vacant designation. Again, depending on the system, this goal can be accomplished with any number of design solutions, from basic clips and holders to high-end electronics. It is appropriate to go beyond simple identification and upgrade areas like boardrooms with graphic elements that make a statement about quality and stability.

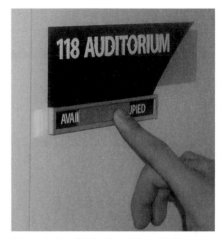

Signage designed by Smallwood, Reynolds, Stewart, Stewart & Associates, Atlanta, for Yamacraw, a Georgia Institute of Technology facility located in Atlanta.

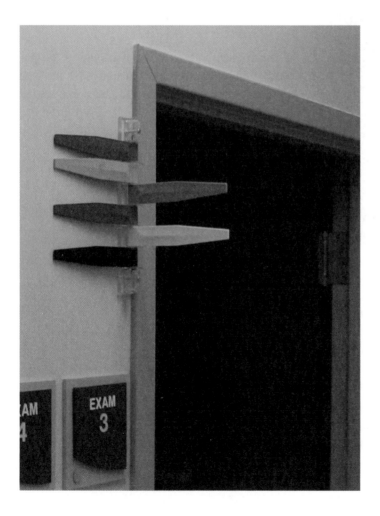

Figure 2-34. Examination Rooms

Examination rooms. In addition to room identification, plaques outside of exam rooms need to communicate a variety of messages to staff, including "in use," "patient in room," and "patient ready to be seen by clinician." Often, hospitals and medical office buildings use a system of color-coded plastic flags mounted at the top of the door frame. (See also chapter 7, figure 7-4.)

Figure 2-35. Patient Care Information/ Chart Boxes

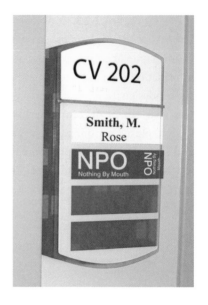

Patient care information/chart boxes. Despite restrictions mandated by the Health Insurance Portability and Accountability Act (HIPAA), some system is needed to display information such as "patient hard of hearing" at the door, and chart boxes often serve the purpose. Such elements may or may not be combined with patient room signage into one module.

Figure 2-36. Restroom Identification

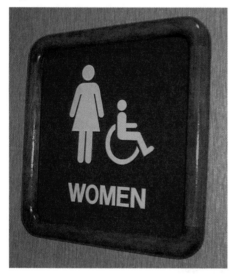

Restroom identification. It is not enough to prominently identify restrooms; you must also indicate whether they are accessible to the handicapped (if not, where should the handicapped go?) and equipped with baby-changing stations (if not, where can one find such a station?). Be aware that unisex designation still gives pause to many people, who feel uncertain about a restroom used by both genders.

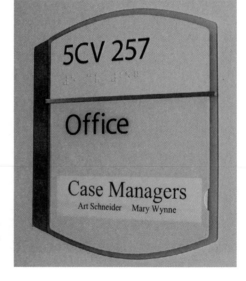

Figure 2-37. Individual Identification

Individual identification. As mentioned earlier in the book, and as will be mentioned again, less is more in signage. However, identification of individuals and the location of that identification are challenges fraught with sensitive issues that each facility must address. Unlike in corporate entities, where the list of key players can be exhaustive, hospitals are more likely to limit individual identification to heads of major departments who are medical doctors.

REGULATORY, POLICY, AND SAFETY SIGNAGE

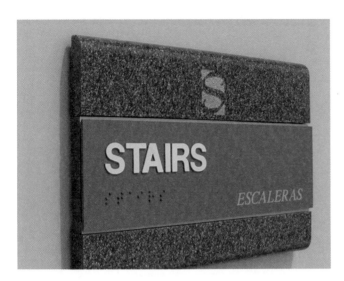

Figure 2-38.
Stairwell Identification

Stairwell and roof access identification. Fire codes require facilities to identify interior and exterior stairwells with specific information and may even dictate a particular-size sign. On the corridor side, the signage must indicate whether the stairs are a viable emergency exit. It may be helpful (or required) to indicate the stairwell number as shown in your life safety files. Interior requirements vary but usually dictate a large image of the floor number and information indicating at what level a visitor can exit and whether roof access is available.

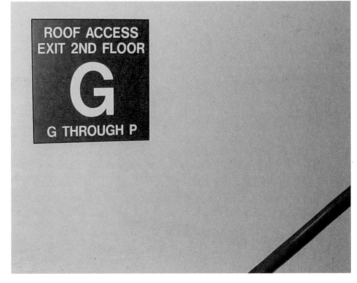

Figure 2-39.
Roof Access Identification

Figure 2-40. Emergency Evacuation Plans

Emergency evacuation plans. Evacuation plans include several components, including floor plans showing where the person is located currently, emergency exit routes, and locations of fire extinguishers and alarms. Keep these signs simple and visually clean—these are not architectural plans—but consider showing areas of rescue and fire doors. If the floor is a large one, break it into wings or quadrants and orient the diagram so that right and left are shown from the viewer's perspective. Finally, get input from the local fire marshal about where to locate the signs.

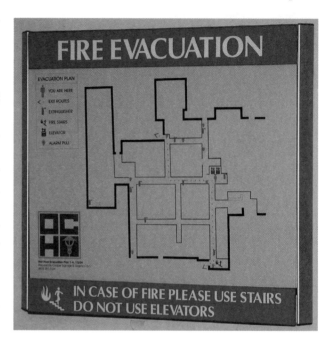

Figure 2-41. Rescue and Disaster Area Signage

Rescue and disaster area signage. Unlike everyday signs, these signs are to be used only on rare occasions and should be kept in a storage closet that is convenient and known to the person responsible for putting them up, as well as her backup. When you need to turn the elevator lobby into a triage station during a crisis, an A-frame sign is ready nearby for use in this situation. Alternatively, a high-definition light-emitting diode (LED) display (figure 2-41) may be put in place that allows shifting from normal use to disaster plan needs with simple command.

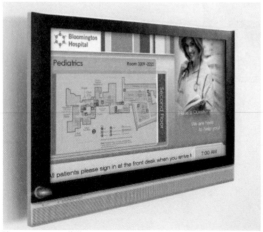

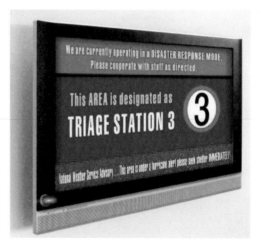

Photos courtesy of Chyron.

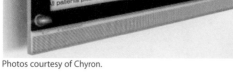

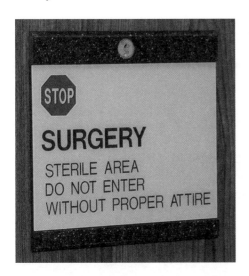

Figure 2-42. Regulatory Signs

Regulatory signs. In addition to U.S. Occupational Safety and Health Administration guidelines and life safety labeling, signage should be provided indicating restricted access or actions in certain areas. This communication involves conveying negative information without seeming negative. For example, the signage may read "Authorized Personnel Only" rather than "Private, Stay Out."

Figure 2-43. Policy Notices

Policy notices. When posting policy notices, you may employ a short way to do this—"This is a tobacco-free facility"—and a long way—"We are concerned about the health of all our visitors, guests, patients, and staff, so please don't smoke. Thank you!" Whichever approach you take, make sure to apply a consistent philosophy to such notices throughout the facility. Remember, readability dramatically improves at seven words or fewer on a sign.

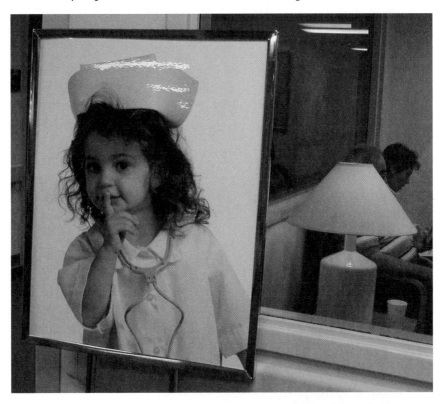

OTHER TYPES OF SIGNAGE IMPORTANT TO WAYFINDING

Figure 2-44. Temporary Informational Signs

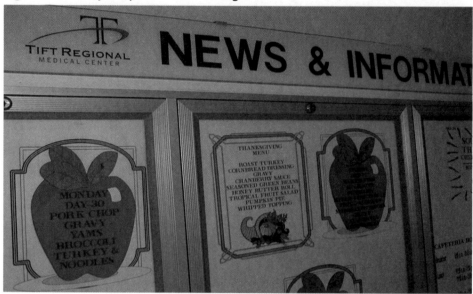

Temporary informational signs. A need will always exist for short-term signs that convey information such as, "Today from 8:00 AM to 10:30 AM, the volunteers will conduct a silent auction in the cafeteria." The key in this signage is to resist complying with each request for such a sign. Determine whether the information is necessary and, if so, where it is needed. Then determine the appropriate size of the sign. Finally, schedule removal

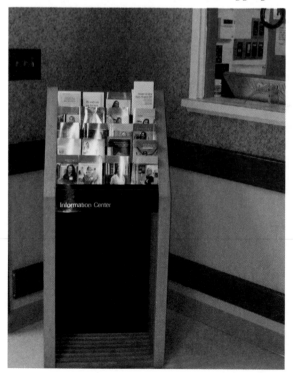

for when the sign will no longer be needed. For the physical requirements of the sign, avoid using exposed push pins, because they can easily fall off an uncovered unit and become a safety hazard. One option is to use grip strips and snap-and-hold frames for quick updates. Electronic signs can also be helpful in this function, which also cut down on visual clutter.

Figure 2-45. Marketing Displays/ Brochure Holder

Marketing displays/brochure holder. Marketing displays need to be monitored and updated frequently. Although many displays are transitioning to high-definition technology, a need to display takeaway brochures and literature will remain for the foreseeable future.

Figure 2-46. Retail/Advertising

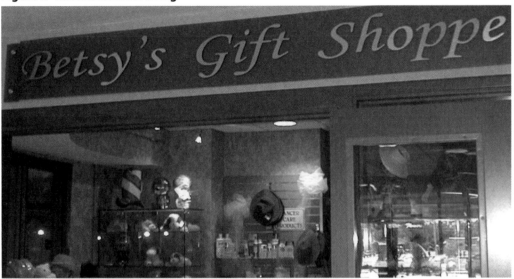

Retail/advertising. Like their exterior counterpart, interior advertising signs are ever more prevalent in hospital areas, from food courts to home care services. These signs require a higher degree of visibility and visual impact but should still fit into the facility's wayfinding lexicon.

Figure 2-47. Dedication/Commemoratory Recognition Signs

Dedication/commemoratory recognition signs. Try to contain the location, size, and quantity of such signs to a limited set. If a donor provides several million dollars to build or upgrade a wing, obviously her name will be placed in more than one prominent spot. For every other donor or subject of commemoration, erecting a central "hall of honor" is a good way to avoid having small signs compete for space and attention haphazardly throughout the facility. Announcement of new programs should be displayed on a limited timeline. Many hospitals tie recognition to the length of a specific fund-raising campaign, at the end of which the names are retired.

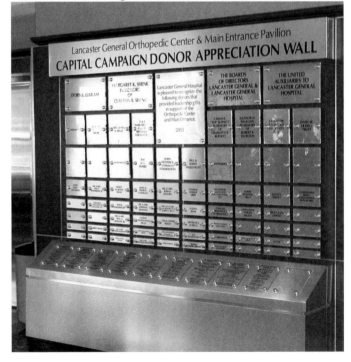

CATCHING UP TO THE DIGITAL AGE

Television now may be viewed on high-definition plasma monitors, information accessed from anywhere in the world via computers, and food orders placed by wait staff on a touch screen device. But we still find our way around the majority of U.S. hospitals using the same static sign systems that have been in place for decades.

Incorporating electronic elements into hospitals' wayfinding system not only facilitates visitors' wayfinding abilities but also projects a strong, high-tech image of their organization to patients and family, community members, and visiting and prospective staff. In addition, electronic signage can support efforts to comply with Americans with Disabilities Act regulations and communicate with non-English-speaking visitors in their own language. The following sections highlight some of the most common technological elements emerging in the health care industry.

GPS Units

Global positioning satellite units are joining printed maps, online map services, and navigational Web sites to help people zero in on their destinations in the hospital. A few facilities are even testing preprogrammed, hand-held GPS units linked to modules concealed in the ceilings along highly trafficked routes. Touch Screen Units

Touch Screen Units

Most commonly used for directories, touch screen units can provide virtual guided tours of specific areas, floors, or buildings—and even print out maps or directions, such as those that one organization, profiled in chapter 8, produced for its main facility and off-site urgent care centers (see figure 2-48). Touch screen applications are ideal for physician referrals because they allow people to search by name, group, specialty, department, or suite number (even accommodating inaccurate or incomplete spelling) and sometimes connect to the Web sites of individual practitioners or clinic facilities. Available options include keyboards, custom screen savers, logos, maps, multilingual capability, audio capability, custom floor plans, maps, and printers. Touch screen units may be housed in desks, walls, or freestanding kiosks. Units can be linked and updated remotely, using off-the-shelf software.

Figure 2-48. Printable Map from Touch Screen Unit

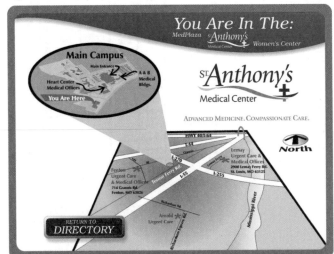

St. Anthony's Medical Center, St. Louis, Missouri, made maps available to visitors through touch screen directories as well as printed visitor guides and Web sites.

Light-Emitting Diode Displays

Figure 2-49. Light-Emitting Diode Displays

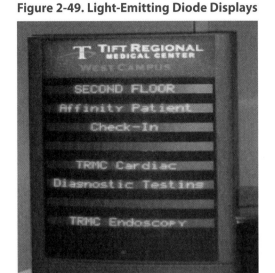

The most common use of LED technology is in exterior site identification signs, often flashing the time and temperature in standard red or amber or, for minimal additional expense, in full color. Inside the facility, LED displays provide an economical way to convey information in multiple languages in a limited space; text can be shown in various colors and fonts, and the message can incorporate pictograms or icons. Easily updated, they might promote a pediatric clinic today and a health fair tomorrow, complete with product tag line or hours of operation. Located in lobbies, they can dissolve from a schedule of daily events and meetings—familiar to visitors of upscale hotels and convention centers—to directory listings to new parking information.

Liquid Crystal Display/Plasma Monitors

Liquid crystal display or plasma monitors bring your message to life in a format that is as user friendly as a television. The only limit to using these units is your imagination. If a hospital wants to provide waiting patients in the emergency room lobby with live TV and also inform them about the Emergency Treatment and Medical Leave Act, HIPAA, and other important policies and rights, a split screen can be used.

Because code inspections lag behind the passage of new codes, and considering each inspector is unique in his knowledge and interpretation of the codes, you may need to duplicate some information with traditional signs. Used to welcome visitors, LCD or plasma monitors can live-feed the time and weather, list daily events, scroll through directories and floor plans, and stream videos developed by the marketing department to promote specific service lines. They can be incorporated into your emergency plans, flashing, for example, "Please keep calm, and evacuate the building" at the stroke of a computer key.

Stationed side by side in transom/soffit-mounted clusters at key decision points and at intervals in long, straight hallways, LCD or plasma units can animate directional messages with arrows, icons, and logos in full-color high definition. Monitors at a cafeteria serving line can feature food choices, prices, and pictures of attractively plated meals; combined with a touch screen kiosk, they can provide nutritional information on demand at no added cost to the organization.

Figure 2-50. Liquid Crystal Display/Plasma Monitors

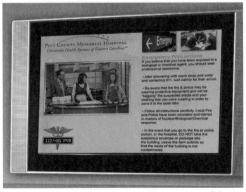

Photo courtesy of Chyron.

Gobo Lights

A gobo is a thin, circular plate with holes cut into it to create patterns of projected light. Used for years in the entertainment industry, gobo lights can highlight a simple logo, graphic, or text by throwing the image onto floors or walls or even exterior walls at night. They may be used to highlight decision points in long hallways or to light an elevator lobby or recessed restrooms.

Returns on Electronic Sign Elements

Hospitals that integrate electronics with solid traditional signage in a well-planned program have reported success based on staff observation and survey results, but adding a single touch screen directory alone provides little return on investment. And it is an investment: Signage is expensive; electronic signage, more so. The need to update equipment renders its usable life to about half that of a fixed system, although the ease of regularly updating information may offset some of the cost over the life of the unit.

Another common pitfall is employing an approach at the other end of the spectrum: loading up on all the possible electronic options for all possible locations to the point where you break the budget. The more complex the setup, the more important it is to buy a maintenance plan and think ahead. One example of anticipating issues that may arise in the future is determining whether updates will occur via hard-wired cables or via wireless, or so-called wi-fi, sensors.

Of course, even the best instruments are only tools in the hands of the musicians. Their value derives from how the tools are used. Electronic displays have great potential as one part of a well-thought-out and well-implemented wayfinding master plan that also includes consistent, user-friendly terminology, comprehensive staff training, accurate maps, and fixed signage working in concert.

UNDERSTANDING THAT PRINT MATERIALS STILL MAKE AN IMPACT

Collateral printed materials can communicate much information at a reasonable cost to the organization. Print materials often include directions, floor plans and maps, organizational policies, phone listings, and answers to frequently asked questions. They are used as auxiliary communication devices that can be posted or put directly into a visitor's hands. Factors to consider regarding the use of print materials include the following:

- The information provided at the time of appointments or appointment reminders must be adequate to ensure the visitor can make the appointment with little effort or anxiety. In addition to indicating the appointment time and department name and location, the flyer or brochure should direct people to a specific parking area, a designated door, and a specific desk at which to register.
- Overly complex or dated maps are worse than no maps. One facility used computer-generated drawings that showed every room and door, resulting in a level of complexity that managed to confuse even insiders.
- If your signs communicate in more than one language, your supportive material should, too.
- Terminology in print materials must be consistent within itself and with signs. You cannot tell people to come to Outpatient Registration and then expect them to know to enter the Day Surgery entrance. Also, use terms that are commonly known to lay visitors. Home Depot does not direct shoppers to aliphatic coating; it directs them to varnishes.

Figure 2-51. Wayfinding with Print Materials

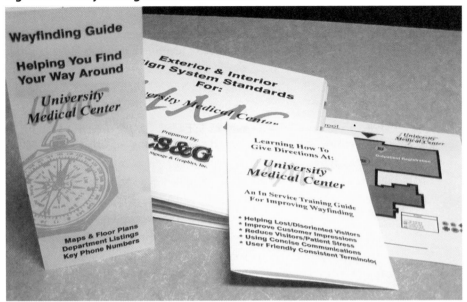

USING ONLINE INFORMATION

As with print materials, it is important to make sure the information (and terminology) provided online is consistent with other communication units and that it is comprehensive. For each destination, the facility's Web site should show patients and visitors where to go, what parking area to use, what door to enter, and the hours during which that entrance is open.

Web sites can be designed as interactive venues, allowing the user to scroll over a site map and a photo of the building. Building name, address, and function all pop up on the interactive map to help visitors become familiar with complex campus settings.

Today, many people use an online map service (such as Google Maps or MapQuest) or GPS to help them get where they are going. Be sure to give a physical street address rather than a central mail drop or post office box for each location on campus.

Hospital Web sites also link clients with off-site clinics, urgent care centers, and other affiliated services, and all of these must be incorporated into the wayfinding plan. If the organization offers online preregistration, either from home or at on-site kiosks, make sure the information requested online is consistent with the in-person registration process. As with any communication tool, attention to the system should not be limited to the initial launch. It is important to keep the sites fresh and up to date.

If Web site access is available at on-site kiosks, make sure the kiosks are designed to be friendly touch screens. Touch screens do not require the same entry precision as does a computer mouse, with which the public is typically more comfortable. Avoid pull-down and drag-and-click items. A kiosk-driven Web site needs to be very basic yet attractive and functional.

KEEPING THE PATIENT IN VIEW

Wayfinding tools combined judiciously, attractively, and consistently into a cohesive whole will nonetheless fail if they do not meet the basic need: getting Pam and Pedro to the right facility at the right time. One way to help keep your wayfinding program responsive to the real world and focused on the patients' experience is to develop a series of typical patient profiles to guide those designing and implementing the program. Consider the two contrasting scenarios that follow.

Pam is a single mother with two young children who has an early-morning appointment on Thursday for a magnetic resonance imaging test (MRI). She will be driving to the hospital, with which she is not familiar. What information does she need to keep that appointment?

- What time to arrive
- The address of the building and how to get there
- Where to park and how much parking will cost (Where should she pay? Does she need a sticker for the windshield? Where does she obtain the sticker?)
- Where to call if she gets lost or is delayed
- What kind of accommodations will be made for the children (and where) if she cannot get a babysitter
- What she should wear and what, if anything, she should bring with her
- How long the procedure (and the wait) will take
- Whether she will be able to drive home unassisted

Depending on the timing, some of this information could be conveyed in a mailed flyer, a reminder phone call (ideally, both), and/or a patient-oriented Web site. But also impor-

tant is to provide the wayfinding clues she will need: What freeway exit should she use? Are trailblazer signs in place to aid her? Is the campus clearly identified and distinguished from the rest of the streetscape? Are the correct parking lot and building entrance for this outpatient procedure clearly labeled? Is a directory or map readily visible to show her how to navigate the building and reach the correct department?

Pedro, also scheduled for an MRI that morning, will be traveling by train from a different part of town entirely and is scheduled for an additional procedure that will require someone to pick him up for his return trip home. He needs to know the following information:

- Which train line to take and which station at which to leave the train
- In which direction to walk from the station to the correct entrance in the correct building (How far is it?)
- Where to have his ride home meet him and when that person should plan to arrive
- Directions for that person to use in driving to the hospital
- Information on where that person is to park and wait if he will need to leave the car and come inside to assist Pedro

It is important to always focus on the experience of the visitor. What seems like an attractive and logical wayfinding system to a hospital committee can only be deemed a success if the number of people who get lost in the hospital is reduced and, ideally, eliminated.

Identifying the Problems and the Players

A comprehensive wayfinding initiative can easily take a year to develop and implement, but it often starts with a single incident. Perhaps a CEO bumps into a visitor in the hallway who has been searching for the cafeteria for 15 minutes. Or a building engineer is called for the third time to replace a "temporary" sign that keeps getting scribbled over and complains to the director of maintenance. Or a patient who has been waiting for 45 minutes to be picked up by her daughter at what turns out to be the wrong exit becomes really angry and calls a hospital board member whom she remembers is married to a co-worker in her office.

Suddenly, a situation that has been quietly deteriorating or taking shape for months, years, or even decades takes on new urgency: Something must be done—now. A staff member—an executive assistant, a marketing staff-person, the "sign guy" who is officially responsible for putting up and taking down signs—is assigned to assess the wayfinding situation.

Perhaps, in a less urgent scenario, the facility is undergoing remodeling to refresh an outdated or worn appearance or to project a new image; perhaps it is growing or being rebuilt to accommodate a new or changing market. Chances are, you are simultaneously working to integrate new regulatory codes and standards and new technology; you may even have a new name or affiliation. Or it may simply be that customer satisfaction surveys combined with anecdotal evidence have revealed a large volume of consistently lost and/or disoriented patients and visitors.

If everyone is thinking alike, then someone isn't thinking. George S. Patton

In any case, you should begin your wayfinding initiative by determining the extent of the problem in your facility. Such a determination can be made through preliminary data gathering. This is round 1 of a general needs assessment.

NEEDS ASSESSMENT, ROUND 1: PRELIMINARY DATA GATHERING

Needs assessment as it relates to wayfinding can run the gamut from talking to colleagues in the cafeteria to hiring professionals to monitor pivotal navigation points—and it usually does. That is, relatively simple steps taken at the start of the assessment can suggest the broad scope

It can't be stressed enough that in order to produce great graphics, you have to have a good product and a good client capable of making decisions. Primo Angeli

and nature of the problem; later, as more people, money, and time are invested into the project, more sophisticated methods will be needed to pinpoint specific issues and generate hard data.

You will want both small, meaningful qualitative data and deeper, verifiable, quantitative statistics to build a foundation for your wayfinding program.

Measuring Customer Satisfaction

Getting a handle on customer satisfaction—or dissatisfaction—is the best place to start.

Track Customer Complaints

Certain people and departments hear the majority of complaints from patients and visitors. These people often are located in areas immediately off elevators and at key decision points along a heavily trafficked pathway. If they are not logging the complaints, they should be. Furthermore, if an individual is not responsible for investigating and responding to those complaints, one should be. Comb through these logs or reports dating back the last several years to discover problems related to wayfinding.

In addition, let staff know that you want to hear when patients and visitors have complaints. From the outset, improved wayfinding is everyone's problem. A panicked visitor stopping a staff member in the hall for directions is an opportunity to create an impression, good or bad. Although it is an often-cited cliché, perception truly becomes reality in this situation: If a visitor feels he received good service, was valued as a consumer, and felt at home in the facility, then he conveys that message to family and friends, who act on or respond to that perception.

Track "Asking for Directions" Encounters

Asking for directions is not always an official complaint, but it should be registered as one.

Staff may assume that giving directions is just an aspect of work life in today's complex facilities and not volunteer the fact that the problem is severe. "I get asked a lot of questions" does not give you much concrete information to work with; "I get asked questions two or three times a day (or a week)" starts to define the problem.

Do not rely on employees' memory for this important count: Give employees a simple log that asks what kind of problem they encountered, where and when it occurred, and how they handled it. Ask employees to keep track of how many wayfinding questions they receive during a predetermined period, typically a week.

When pressed to give a quantity to the problem, one large facility could not do so; it defaulted to a response of "a lot." But when a log was kept, staff in the facility found in a week's time that 290 people were searching for an obscure entrance. That count was an important factor in motivating the administration to address the problem area.

Conduct Satisfaction Surveys

Chances are, your hospital already surveys patients and visitors to determine their satisfaction, perhaps via a follow-up phone call or letter. If so, especially if the survey includes open-ended questions about the individual's experience, these surveys may yield interesting data just waiting to be gleaned, in comments such as "I always felt like I was walking in circles" or "It took forever to find X-Ray."

Incorporating targeted questions about wayfinding into the standard survey will generate more—and more useful—information in short order. Your marketing department either has or can access professional expertise in structuring questions that will yield productive answers. For example, "Were you able to easily get where you needed to be during your recent visit?" "How hard was it to find your way around ABC facility on your recent visit?"

Other ways of obtaining this information can be used to augment the standard customer survey, including the following:

- Pull together a focus group of recent patients and visitors to explore their experiences. This step signals to the community that the organization values the public's input and that supporting the concept of patient and family care is a consideration throughout the facility's operations.
- Call on the opinions of community groups that already have a relationship with the organization. These groups could include disabled veterans to help identify problems with accessibility, or senior citizens from a nursing home (perhaps as a test group) to determine how the elderly respond to finding their way around your facility.
- Set up a sampling station at an exit point or in the parking lot for persons who volunteer to answer questions, verbally or in a printed survey, on the spot. (No soliciting, please—you do not want to hassle worried, anxious, or ill people.)

Additional Data Collection Techniques

Described below are other data collection techniques you can use at this early stage to supplement your complaint system and customer satisfaction queries.

Review Industry Data

A recent survey conducted by the American Hospital Association (AHA) and the author's firm revealed that 74 percent of facilities had recently reviewed their wayfinding needs, and 61 percent indicated that their wayfinding was not up to date. The same survey showed that only 56 percent of facilities provide any form of map or visitor guide. (See the 2008 Wayfinding Needs Survey conducted by the AHA's Society for Healthcare Strategy and Market Development and AHA Solutions.[1]) Other health care industry statistics have shown that lost staff time, reduced revenue due to adjusting schedules, and lower customer satisfaction are just a few problems associated with poor wayfinding.[2]

In another survey by the AHA, more than 50 percent of all facilities reported that a lack of adequate wayfinding in their facilities had created significant problems. In addition, the report states, "According to the findings, the overwhelming majority of U.S. health care executives (89 percent) reveal their facility has poor patient flow."[3] Data revealed by these and other surveys of the industry will help you understand the problems in your own organization.

Review Organizational Plans

If you have a master facility plan, you still have time to start planning for how projected changes or additions will affect your wayfinding program. Likewise, wayfinding programs will need to be in synch with the organization's strategic planning and marketing goals and timetables. Perhaps the organization is planning to introduce new service lines or products in the next two years—a women's care pavilion, say, or an orthopedic center. Do not adopt a signage system today that will not work well with what the organization will look like—in terms of physical structure and, just as important, image—in two or five years. A system that is difficult to update will not be current for long, and any system that does not properly communicate inflicts more damage to patient care, visitor satisfaction, and public image than it promotes good service.

Similarly, if the organization is planning for a new technology platform that will allow the use of high-definition television as part of a signage system, be ready to take advantage of that opportunity.

Conduct a Visual Inspection

Are your signs, maps, and directories inconsistent, referring to the outpatient laboratory as Outpatient Testing on one sign and to Laboratory at another? Are the signs fading? Do the colors scream 1980s at a time when you are competing with a brand-new hospital in the area? Does the signage system meet current codes and standards, or are they two generations behind?

Are signs well placed? Or is the directory located behind the reception desk, where people cannot see or access it?

Are materials outdated? Is ad hoc paper signage taped up everywhere—or, indeed, anywhere—inconsistent with your image as a quality provider and technology leader?

(A favorite example: a restroom sign reading "Restroom is broken, please use floor below.")

You can easily create visual pollution when you start with hundreds or thousands of official signs, handouts, brochures, and collateral pieces and then allow physicians, specialty groups, and departments to generate their own without having a process in place to review them for accuracy and appropriateness. Are those proliferating additions up to date, concise, attractive, and consistent?

A different kind of visual pollution results when succeeding generations of designers, each with her own agenda, quickly erect signs that may answer a current need but clash with older signage. Look for instances of "oversigning," that is, signage that evolves over time

Figure 3-1. Visual Pollution

A highly public pharmacy window at one urban hospital serves hundreds of patients daily. Imagine their confusion when confronted with so many messages.

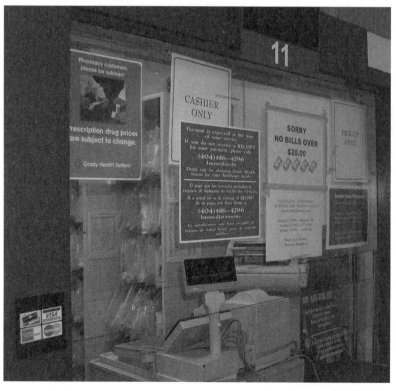

from multiple requests and ends up creating visual pollution (figure 3-1).

Years ago, signs may simply have read, "Smoking in designated areas only." Later, "Healing place—no smoking" signs were put up. When facilities state- or citywide were mandated to be smoke-free environments, "This is a tobacco-free campus" signs joined the fray. Many hospitals have not removed the previous generations of signs, making it possible for smokers to choose to obey the message they prefer, or to simply ignore them all.

Commission Independent Surveys

Custom design your on-site surveys to determine how a visitor experiences the physical facility. Survey questions for a one-story, 100-bed hospital will be dramatically different from those directed to a 1,200-bed complex with multiple support buildings and clinics. Conduct random intercept interviews of visitors to determine problem areas. This information is small in sample, but it will provide good qualitative data on which to build or update your wayfinding program.

As you delve deeper into the question of visitor experience, conduct staff interviews (in person or online) to widen your database and render it more quantitative and verifiable. In a facility expansion program, for example, you would focus efforts on the departments relocating into the new area and those moving into the old spaces. In a new or replacement facility, the interviews may need to be directed toward every department head. Engineering, marketing, nursing services, volunteer services, and administration should be surveyed in just about every case. Once the information is gathered, follow-up discussions of specific concepts to address particular needs are helpful to make sure solutions hit their targets.

Figure 3-2 contains a survey tool for staff to self-diagnose wayfinding problems, expanding your database further. The tool can be used to help identify your facility's specific strengths and weaknesses, giving you a solid foundation on which to develop a wayfinding program that is sensitive to the current situation and adaptable to changes in the future. (And there *will* be changes.)

Once the initial fact-finding measures have yielded a general impression of the problems you face, and once these have been compiled into a preliminary report, it is time to dig deeper. This is no longer a one- or two-person job. You need a team to conduct the next phase of needs assessment.

TEAM BUILDING

Every facility compiles a project committee or task force based on its own needs and talents. This team should include a core group of people who have the interest and time to invest over the long term, as well as others who are asked to join at and for specific phases of the project. As a group, the committee may wish to reach out to a wayfinding design consultant, who can help it define and refine a program that will meet the organization's specific needs.

No hard and fast rules dictate who should serve, but it will be hard to carry out the necessary work of the committee with fewer than four or more than twelve members in the core group.

Candidates for Committee Membership

The following areas and disciplines are excellent places to look for wayfinding committee members:

- Administration
- Engineering/building and grounds services

Figure 3-2. Wayfinding Audit Checklist

Facility Surveyed _____

Conducted by _____ Date of Survey _____

On a scale of 1 to 5, please indicate the degree to which the following statements apply to your facility.

1 = strongly disagree
2 = disagree
3 = could go either way
4 = agree
5 = strongly agree

_____   We have significant numbers of patients routinely needing directions.

_____   It has been more than 5 years since we last evaluated our approach to wayfinding.

_____   Our signage does not reflect the desired image.

_____   Our signage is inconsistent in appearance.

_____   Our signage is not easy and economical to maintain or add to.

_____   We do not have a sign system manual.

_____   Our signs do not have tactile text and Grade II Braille.

_____   Our signs address only English speakers.

_____   Our signs present visual clutter.

_____   Staff is not trained on how to give directions.

_____   We use inconsistent terminology for destinations, both verbally and in signage.

_____   We do not have an easy-to-use map of the campus and outlying destinations.

_____   We do not provide complete campus information at physicians' offices and on the web.

_____   We do not have a comprehensive, facility-wide room numbering system.

_____   Our signage does not distinguish among elevators.

_____   It is unclear which entrance is to be used at what times or for which needs.

_____   We have a new logo, name, or affiliation.

_____   We have significantly expanded since our last wayfinding audit/review.

_____   We want to project a fresher image to the community.

_____   Subtotal

_____   Add 5 points if you are expanding/renovating

_____   TOTAL

Total possible points: 100

If you amass more than 50, you probably need to update or implement a comprehensive wayfinding plan. However, any one "strongly agree" item may point to a serious enough problem for you to consider reconfigured or additional wayfinding components or approaches.

- Information technology
- Admitting
- Nursing
- Marketing and communications
- Translation services
- Business office
- Food services
- Volunteer services
- The organization's foundation
- Physicians
- Purchasing and materials management

Below we consider them one by one, starting with the senior-level management, or C-suite.

Administration. Administration must buy into the idea of providing a comprehensive wayfinding system, dedicated to improving patient throughput and satisfaction. With limited time available, the hospital or health system's top leaders will probably not chair the group or even attend every committee meeting. However, they do need regular two-way communication with the group, and a representative from or with the ear of the C-suite should head the effort at least until the plan has taken shape. Often the person in this role is the chief operating officer (COO) or the director of engineering.

Engineering/building and grounds services. Charged with the thankless job of keeping the entire campus fresh and well maintained, these are the people on everyone's speed dial. Their perspective and involvement are essential in establishing viable parameters for the program and in its successful implementation. As the "go-to" group that updates the building(s), it knows the expansion and renovation schedules and should always be considered part of the wayfinding team. After the initial wayfinding committee disbands, the engineering department may be used to relocate, take down, and update both interior and exterior signs. As such, its staff need to know the overall intent of the signage; the standards required for creating the signs; and details such as proper sign mounting, removal, and storage.

Information technology. What scheme will work with the organization's current and anticipated hardware and software, and what issues might interfere with the systems in use? The information technology department will make sure the committee is headed down a clear path.

Admitting. Policies, procedures, and staffing levels will affect who needs to go where and when. Some facilities use entrance A for admitting from 6 AM to 8 AM, entrance B from 8 AM to 5 PM, then the emergency department entrance from 5 PM to 6 AM. The questions are, how is this information communicated, and how likely is it to change? Signage details—such as the hours of operation for a new service or for an entrance or check-in desk—may need to be adjusted several times until proper staffing levels are determined. The admitting staff can ensure that the signs are changed in response to this need.

Nursing. Understaffed and overworked, nurses do not need to add "guide" to their job description. The way patients and visitors experience the organization is one of nursing's top priorities, and effective wayfinding frees caregivers to focus on caregiving.

Marketing and communications. As guardians of the corporate brand and standards, identity, and image, these departments have a huge stake in seeing that signage does its part to promote individual products and services, including those off-campus components that can feel like stepchildren, along with the facility as a whole.

Translation services. For people whose English cannot be relied on to give or receive crucial medical information, the last thing they need is to get lost in your facility. This department is responsible for ensuring that the wayfinding program works to get limited English proficiency visitors where they need to go, quickly and safely.

Business office. Like many nonclinical spaces, the business office may be located where the facility has space available for this purpose, but not necessarily in a location with the best access to the public. The organization's revenue stream flows through this office, so wayfinding procedures, policies, and signage need to work together to ensure patients have easy access to this important department.

Food services. As well as a source of welcome sustenance to anxious people (who are not the captive audience they use to be), the facility's cafeterias, snack bars, and coffee shops are, ideally, also profit centers. Ask anyone who owns a restaurant whether it is important that their clients be able to locate them, navigate the menu, and get the food they want when they want it. Food service personnel recognize they are in the restaurant business along with serving patients in their rooms. Promoting sales is part of that reality: The old adage that you sell the sizzle, not the steak, is just as true in hospitals, and signage (especially high-definition displays) can promote product sales. Additionally, food service signage can display health information to promote wellness programs to visitors and staff.

Volunteer services. Volunteers are often the first representatives of the organization whom visitors encounter. They are helpers by nature: If not properly trained in the art of giving directions, they will use their own method—sometimes good, sometimes bad, rarely consistent. They also are a great grassroots resource for identifying problems in patient flow.

The foundation. Chances are, your hospital seriously needs the funding and community support its foundation provides. That means your wayfinding program will need to recognize donors. Involving foundation staff will ensure that donor recognition messages honor the donors gracefully without undercutting program standards.

Physicians. This contingent is the real lifeblood of your facility. Physicians are known to have opinions and share comments on every aspect of the hospital, so give them a constructive method by which to provide their input. If you get key physicians engaged, the whole program takes on a higher profile.

Purchasing and materials management. A carefully devised plan that cannot be implemented is worse than useless, which is why the individuals in this area are so important to the wayfinding effort. Purchasing will have a lot to say about how the program is implemented and what cost center will pay for it, while materials management will need to contribute its resources and expertise in procurement. Astute buyers understand that wayfinding elements are not off-the-shelf commodities. For example, they may employ in-house printers to keep up on forms, letterhead, and such, but they may have higher priorities than updating your visitors guide or floor plan. The materials management staff also will realize that the old practice of bidding signage will not necessarily work well in this context: If investigating a request and issuing a purchase order take four to five weeks, every out-of-date sign will stay up that much longer. Establishing a standard price list, blanket purchase orders, and a strong relationship with a reliable source can streamline the process significantly.

Common Pitfalls in Team Building

Team building is fraught with perils. Take heed to avoid these common pitfalls:

- Getting the wrong people, or not enough people, involved

Examples: failing to engage the C-suite, talking only to complainers, expecting one person to do all the needs assessment, waiting for staff to volunteer

- Not pulling the team together early enough to capitalize on the initial interest/need
Examples: waiting until a very visible crisis occurs to act, not meeting frequently enough, not assigning specific tasks to individuals, not setting deadlines
- Poorly defining, or overly restricting, the scope of the project
Examples: focusing only on the interior when getting people in the right door is more than half the battle, limiting the scope to new construction and not dealing with existing spaces

These pitfalls can be avoided with strong project leadership and committee-to-committee linkages.

Project Leadership

Your project needs both a committee chair and a project manager; in all likelihood, these roles are played by two different people. Again, the chair needs to either be in the C-suite or have direct access to it in order to deal effectively with the politics of the situation, set direction, and identify funding sources. She is therefore unlikely to have the time or manual skills to be the hands-on, go-to person. Someone else needs to step forward and agree to be the "sign person"—the program champion, liaison to department heads, or continuity manager.

So if, for example, the COO or director of purchasing takes the helm at the start and sees the project through the planning and design development phases, he will probably ask someone else to pick up the reins for the implementation of those plans and designs—maybe a member of maintenance or housekeeping, for example. This individual is your project manager.

Keep in mind that the project manager is the person whom everyone will call—forever—when a new sign is needed and who will have to tell the unit secretary on 3E why she cannot have her name on that sign. So this must be someone who knows how to get things done and works well with others: a doer and a diplomat.

Committee-to-Committee Linkages

Your committee will want to have strong working links to other committees with related concerns. These linkages can be forged through periodic invitations to attend each other's meetings, designation of official liaisons, regular reports, and/or overlapping appointments. Groups that might make an important contribution to the wayfinding initiative include the following standing committees:

- Customer satisfaction
- Patient throughput
- Safety

Customer satisfaction committee. It is the job of this group to step back and see the facility as outsiders see it. "Outsiders" include not just patients and their families but also a broad spectrum of customers: visiting clinicians, current and potential employees, and community representatives, among others. Is ease of navigating your facility a factor in their satisfaction, or dissatisfaction? Just ask them.

Patient throughput committee. The members of this committee may equal or exceed your enthusiasm for getting patients to their procedures on time; every time a piece of expensive equipment sits idle or a staff schedule is disrupted because a patient is running late, the failure is theirs. It is to their advantage to make sure your wayfinding program starts *before* that patient arrives at the facility. For example, the reminder phone call the day before a person's appointment as well as the preadmission package that gets mailed can easily include directions about which entrance to enter, where to park, and how to find the examination room.

Safety committee. "Don't leave valuables in your car." "Emergency call button." "Call the front desk for an escort." These are just a few examples of the intersection of wayfinding and safety concerns. The people serving on this committee can help you identify others and suggest ways to make the environment safer for everyone.

CHOOSING A WAYFINDING DESIGN CONSULTANT

So far, so good. But while all these people are professionals in managing aspects of health care, they may not have the expertise to manage aspects of wayfinding. A wayfinding design consultant is an individual designer or a firm with knowledge of the processes needed to develop and implement a sound wayfinding program. An experienced wayfinding design consultant knows industry standards, is familiar with the available technology, and understands the trends in wayfinding.

The committee should ensure that the design consultant has experience in health care wayfinding. Furthermore, it should look for a consultant who has worked with similar kinds of facilities, whether a rural community clinic or an urban teaching hospital.

This same tenet applies to implementation. The processes of value engineering, meeting deadlines, and creating products that work and also promote the organization's mission and image are comparable to walking a tightrope. Again, there is no substitute for appropriate experience.

That said, do not take a design consultant's word that she has obtained that experience. Ask to see documentation, get the names of former clients with whom you may speak, and get pictures of—or better yet, visit—the client facilities.

A Three-Step Selection Process

Before selecting a design consultant, you will need to perform your due diligence and seek qualifications from several companies, then short-list two or three for full tours and in-depth interviews.

First, the committee should look through buyers guides, perform Web searches, and ask colleagues inside and outside the organization—particularly those at facilities whose wayfinding program you admire—for referrals. This inquiry process will likely uncover a wide range of design consultants who are eager to help. A comprehensive request for proposal (RFP) process will help narrow the list to those with appropriate credentials. (See appendix A for a sample RFP.)

An RFP should include the following items:

- An overview of the facility, including any off-site locations, affiliates, or other related facilities.
- Wayfinding problems you want addressed (attach the preliminary report created in the step described earlier).
- Schedule requirements, referencing any current or proposed construction/ renovation projects.
- The response format you prefer, including written versus personal presentation, number of copies to be submitted, and in what format.
- The criteria the committee will use in selecting the successful candidate.
- Contract details, or terms and conditions (e.g., payment schedule, timeline, duration of contract).
- Background information required.

- Detailed costs associated with the scope of services, including expenses and any optional service. Some additional services might include focus group testing, patient survey administration, filing for variances, and dealing with a host of potential surprises, including (1) applying for the sign permit and being turned down, requiring extensive redesign (who pays for these adjustments?); (2) changing the scope of the project, even slightly (how does this take place, what cost is involved, and who handles it?); or (3) building on the original wayfinding concept through a new expansion a year later (how does this take place, and what fees are involved from the consultant?). Identify these services up front to control the project.
- References.

Second, the finalists will each need a comprehensive tour of your facility, highlighting the problem areas you have identified and possible solutions that have been suggested by staff. If necessary, this tour can be conducted with the potential vendors all at one time, but better results will be achieved if the tours are conducted on a one-on-one basis, as long as each consultant receives the same basic information. In solo tours, each candidate will be compelled to give her honest assessment and best ideas rather than be swayed by hints from other candidates about their proposal. If different members of the committee conduct the tours, each should operate using the same talking points.

Similarly, the interviews should be conducted one-on-one. Although it is more time consuming to talk with each candidate on the short list separately, resist the temptation to hold a group question-and-answer session; this format does not allow for the same depth or degree of intimacy as individual meetings.

Each vendor will want the opportunity to ask questions and sell his approach separately, and this expectation is certainly reasonable as long as no upfront fee is involved and staff have the time to conduct the interviews.

Allow two to four weeks for a written proposal to be submitted by candidates, with minimal supportive literature or boilerplate copy. A good method for communicating what will be meaningful to your selection team is to spell out clearly what respondents should and should not include in their package. For example, project portfolios of casinos as clients may make nice presentations but are of little value to your organization.

Third, the committee will need to choose a vendor. You may want to develop a scoring or ranking system to help you make the final selection. In the end, assuming more than one affordable vendor is willing and able to do the job, whom you will be most comfortable working with is a gut-level decision. Keep in mind that you are not hiring this consultant to meet short-term financial or logistical concerns; you are, ideally, forming a lasting partnership.

Knowing Your Sign Company: Whom Are You Signing Up?

To the general public, a sign is a sign is a sign— and a sign company makes signs, period. Your wayfinding committee needs to recognize that the process is more complex than this superficial concept implies. It needs to know that the historical line between architectural and commercial signage firms—the first producing sophisticated, systems-oriented, and highly aesthetic interior signs to project a corporate image, the latter producing large exterior signs designed to generate business—has been blurred ever since small companies began to specialize in installing both kinds of signs in the 1980s and 1990s. In many states, all that is needed to install a sign is a pickup truck and a ladder.

In the mid-1980s, the advent of vinyl-cutting equipment spawned the "quick sign" business, which featured quick and basic planning on the side. Fighting this trend, some leading West Coast sign firms began offering planning services as well, often at a fraction of the price charged by traditional design firms. In response, the traditional design firms decided to sell their own signs and throw in value-added retail services they either offer themselves or broker.

So just whom are you dealing with—a design firm that provides signs? A sign firm that provides design? Or an architectural sign company that is knowledgeable and experienced in both? We strongly recommend the last.

> Take Note. Two approaches may be used to bring in outside expertise for a wayfinding project: In the *design-bid-build* approach, the design consultant signs off on the project and turns it over to the sign company that will actually fabricate and install the physical signs. In the *design-build* approach, the design consultant completes the entire project itself. See chapter 5 for a discussion of the design-bid-build versus the design-build approach.

NEEDS ASSESSMENT, ROUND 2: DIGGING DEEPER

Once your full wayfinding program team is working together, the final round of needs assessment should be conducted, this time using specific measures to evaluate performance and return on investment as the initiative moves forward. The measures are developed to quantify and qualify the impressions and ideas gathered in the first round

and to track progress toward desired goals as they become clearer to the wayfinding committee. (See chapter 4 for discussions of goal setting and performance criteria.) If hired, a wayfinding design consultant takes the lead at this point, starting with a subjective review of the facility and ending with preparation of the final report—including plenty of photographs as evidence of issues needing to be addressed—for the committee to approve. For example, the consultant may state in the report, "Current signage is not a single unified system in appearance, creating a visually cluttered environment" and include a photo illustrating an area in which several signs are different in appearance and fight for visual dominance.

The consultant's report states the obvious problems that go unobserved on a daily basis, such as duplicate signs or signs with conflicting messages, and brings each team member into alignment with the stage of the process. The final report, shared with all staff, will enlist employees to learn to spot visual pollution, identify problems and a final target for the wayfinding initiative, and begin to understand how to correct these situations. The visual report is also a good before-and-after study to review project results at a later date.

In preparing the report, the design consultant should use some or all of the following approaches:

- Review all relevant printed materials.
- Conduct in-depth staff interviews.
- Monitor hot spots and decision points.
- Arrange or lead site visits.

See chapter 4 for more detail on the consultant's report, which serves as one of several control documents guiding the wayfinding project.

Reviewing All Relevant Printed Materials

Relevant printed materials include the facility's visitors guide, maps, procedure-specific brochures, and any other items that include wayfinding information. Are there too many? Too few? Do they address special circumstances such as weekend and after-hours status? Is the terminology consistent? Are the messages on target and up to date? Are they translated into languages commonly spoken in the community? Is the text sexist? Ageist? Confusing?

Conducting In-Depth Staff Interviews

While initial surveys provide an overview of the needs, deeper interviews allow insight into specific problem areas identified in the initial survey. Statistical data will never be able to replace face-to-face interviews with key staff members or directors in such areas as nursing, engineering, marketing, purchasing, admitting/registration, and volunteer services. These interviews will show staff that wayfinding improvements are a priority with the administration. Another advantage of in-depth interviews is the opportunity it provides to introduce wayfinding concepts that will later be instituted with in-service training, such as training on the art of giving directions (see chapter 5, "Implementation").

To supplement the in-depth interviews with key staff, you can schedule open forums to allow those who have additional concerns to discuss them, even if they are not targeted for input by the team. It is critical to let everyone know that these meetings are for gleaning information and that they will not necessarily be involved in future presentations of possible solutions. Last, these forums will pave the way for a larger buy-in of the final wayfinding program at all levels.

A number of ways are available to interview a wide range of staff members. You can have a big staff meeting and throw open the floor to anyone who wants to bring up a problem for discussion. Or you can set up a meeting room for two to three days and schedule appointments every 15 or 30 minutes. In the latter format, staff members enter one at a time and explain where they work and what they do. ("Hi, I'm Earl Garrett. I'm head of building services and I work in 3E. I'll be in the new tower when it's completed.")

To each interviewee, the design consultant ought to pose the same questions: What are your problems? Why can't people find you? Who is looking for you, and what are their concerns? The answers will often be surprising. In the process of interviewing staff at South Georgia Medical Center, a rural Southern hospital, for example, a design consultant discovered that, although the translation services department had documented a user rate of just 4 percent, nurses reported through an on-site survey (conducted by the author's firm in 2008 at the medical center) that Spanish-only speakers made up about a quarter of all customers. Why hadn't the nurses requested help? Because it would generate additional paperwork, and it was easier to simply enlist the help of bilingual friends, family members, or staff members.

The more people who are feeding information into the needs assessment process, the better, as long as that input is organized, timely, and relevant to the wayfinding improvement process.

The best way to ensure maximum buy-in from the maximum number of people is to give everyone with something to say a chance to say it—and to actually listen to each person. Even people with no expertise or authority have an opinion about a concept as basic as wayfinding, and if the program you design does not respect their opinion, those people will not like it, period.

Furthermore, you *need* that input. When it comes to navigating your facility and helping others to do the same, a cafeteria worker probably has more experience than a senior vice president who rarely leaves the C-suite. You want both to embrace the wayfinding program with equal enthusiasm.

Monitoring Hot Spots and Decision Points

You can learn a lot simply by posting a trained observer at key spots, such as elevator lobbies, building directories, and laboratories, to watch how visitors behave. Do they hesitate? Backtrack? Turn around in bewildered circles? This kind of monitoring is best done by the design consultant or an outside firm she hires, but it can also be very revealing to augment the process by bringing in lay volunteers, assigning each to a specific location, and debriefing them afterward about their experience.

Hot spots and decision points can be monitored on an ongoing basis. For example, this process should be repeated as a testing procedure after a beta series of directional signs is placed in a given environment (see "Rollout and Phasing" in chapter 5). The process will enable you or your consultant to observe whether new wayfinding elements have had the desired impact.

Arranging or Leading Site Visits

How does your facility fare in comparison with the local and regional competition? To get an idea of what other, similar kinds of facilities are doing, make sure the design consultant takes the wayfinding committee (or individual members) on site visits: Take plenty of pictures and talk with the people who were involved in developing and implementing the wayfinding program. Are they pleased with their solutions? What problems have they encountered? What would they do differently if they were starting over?

Bring back all the information and feed it into the planning process—which you are now ready to start.

REFERENCES

1. Cooper Signage & Graphics for Society for Healthcare Strategy and Market Development (SHSMD) and AHA Solutions, "Wayfinding Needs of Health Care Facilities." Needs Determination Series. Chicago: SHSMD and AHA Solutions, 2008.

2. StatCom, "2008 National Survey on Patient Flow Challenges and Technologies," Alpharetta, GA: StatCom.

3. American Hospital Association (AHA), "2009 Patient Flow Challenges Assessment," Chicago: AHA, 2009.

CHAPTER 4

Planning and Designing

Having assembled your committee, enlisted professional help, and completed your needs assessment, you are now ready to plan your wayfinding project. This phase of the total process includes setting goals; establishing further performance criteria, budgets and timelines, and design development; and preparing documentation.

Together, these activities will generate your organization's wayfinding program. Remember, this process is more than just hanging signs. It deals with elements such as corporate branding, product positioning, code compliance, and utilitarian communications (e.g., "Patients will be seen in order of medical need, not in order of arrival") that identify, communicate, inform, and restrict.

> The designer does not, as a rule, begin with a preconceived idea. His idea is the result of subjective and objective thought, and the design a product of the idea. In order, therefore, to achieve an honest and effective solution he necessarily passes through some sort of mental process. . . . Consciously or not, he analyzes, interprets, translates. . . . He improvises, invents new techniques and combinations. He coordinates and integrates his material so that he may restate his problem in terms of ideas, pictures, forms, and shapes. He unifies, simplifies, and eliminates superfluities. He symbolizes . . . abstract from his material by association and analogy. He intensifies and reinforces his symbol with appropriate accessories to achieve clarity and interest. He draws upon instinct and intuition. He considers the spectator, his feelings and predilections. Paul Rand

COMMON PITFALLS IN PLANNING

At the outset, your committee should be aware of potential pitfalls in the planning process. The following list includes those that are most common.

Using unqualified consultants or those with limited expertise. For example:

- Hiring an architect who specializes in upscale hotels rather than health care facilities
- Hiring a contractor new to the industry to save money
- Asking a maintenance worker to design landscaping to reinforce the corporate image

Not establishing a viable working budget early in the process. For example:

- Allowing expectations to surpass what the organization can ultimately afford
- Failing to allocate enough money to complete all phases of implementation
- Budgeting less money than is realistic to meet committee expectations

Failing to plan for expansion/upkeep. For example:

- Not establishing a timetable for updating printed materials and signage
- Using the standard ordering process instead of a streamlined process that is in synch with in-house capabilities
- Choosing materials and techniques without factoring in a rise in costs over time

Overcommunicating. For example:

- Using too many signs or too many words, as when listing all office tenants, payment policies, hours, and logos on one sign or erecting separate signs for each occupant in a shared suite.

Relying on signs to meet every need. For example:

- Putting up a sign in response to every question or complaint
- Assuming that all people read signs

Not checking local codes/permitting processes. For example:

- Ignoring codes and inspectors
- Not documenting your processes in case of disputes

Selecting colors from small chips away from the affected environment. For example:

- Assuming that a color will look the same inside and outside without checking
- Not checking the color under natural or artificial light, whichever will be its setting
- Agreeing to go "two shades darker" without seeing the actual color in question

A wayfinding program not only deals with the facility or campus as it currently exists but also looks ahead to future growth and the inevitable changes that make the industry so dynamic. Having a progressive plan in place will allow you to avoid another common pitfall experienced in so many aspects of health care: responding in reflexive fashion to change without having time to maintain a high level of quality and, in this case, aesthetics. Progressive planning begins with setting goals.

SETTING GOALS

The following sentence is a broad statement of purpose: "Memorial Hospital seeks to improve the visitor and patient experience, reduce stress, enhance aesthetics, and improve efficiency through updated wayfinding." Such a statement is a good place to start in the goal-setting process and can help introduce the rest of the organization to the activities and rationale of the wayfinding committee—and the organization will want to know both before giving you its full cooperation.

Beyond articulating a statement of purpose, you will need to focus your efforts on plausible solutions for achieving your goals (figure 4-1). Traditional concepts (scenario 1)

Figure 4-1. Scenarios for Achieving Your Goals
Many great ideas can be offered, but focus your efforts on plausible solutions to complete the project.

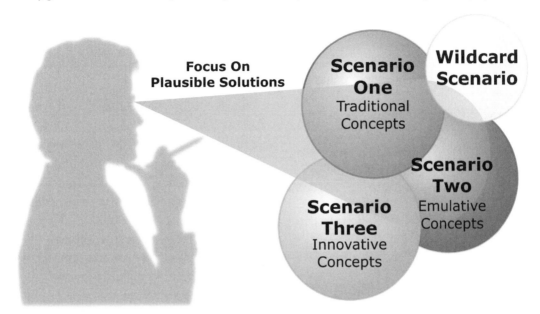

are simply those you have applied in the past, which build on what works and modify or discard what has not worked. Emulative concepts (scenario 2) take ideas from other facilities' efforts and incorporate them into your solutions. (Sometimes reinventing the wheel is simply not needed to achieve your goals.) Innovative concepts (scenario 3) introduce an element that does not have a proven history but, based on solid research and careful development, will bring value to the project that may not be available from more proven concepts.

Wild-card scenarios are best thought of as "way outside the box" thinking—solutions for which facilities are prepared to pave the way and take some risk. These can be as simple as radically new color combinations or as wild as giving every visitor a handheld telemetry device to personalize his wayfinding experience. Wild-card scenarios are a designer's dream and can result in big rewards.

Focusing on plausible solutions does not exclude innovation. In fact, by examining all scenarios, you will focus on creative solutions that stand apart from the others. The point is to know where you are heading and why.

A statement of purpose and a focus on plausible solutions can help you consider how much you want the facility to resemble other similar places, or how much originality you hope to achieve. But a statement of purpose and plausible solutions are not sufficient to guide your program planning and its eventual implementation. You also need more specific and, just as important, measurable goals that address the particular problems or areas of concern you have identified. The data you gathered during the needs assessment process (chapter 3) can serve as a baseline, allowing you to quantify improvement.

Designers can create normalcy out of chaos; they can clearly communicate ideas through the organizing and manipulating of words and pictures. Jeffery Veen

Following are some often-used goals you may want to take on or adapt for your own project:

- Fewer customer complaints
- Higher customer satisfaction scores
- Fewer requests for directions registered by staff
- Fewer staff requests for new or replacement signs
- Fewer staff requests for sign maintenance
- Better on-time registration rates for outpatient procedures and tests

In addition, you can, and should, score the performance of the design consultant, other vendors that may be brought in, and responsible staff in carrying out their assigned tasks according to predetermined criteria.

But what kind of criteria?

ESTABLISHING PERFORMANCE CRITERIA OR PARAMETERS

Here, again, every organization must identify for itself an appropriate set of criteria or parameters to guide the parties during the wayfinding project. Many of these criteria will apply primarily to the design process, but others will have implications for sign installers, maintenance staff, budget developers, and others.

These criteria should be established jointly by the committee with the design consultant. Following are some fruitful areas for discussion:

- User group demographics
- Applicable codes and standards
- Financial constraints
- Quality
- Overall aesthetic tone

User Group Demographics

At all decision points in the planning process, the perspective of the patient and visitor should be your guide. Whether you use color coding, facility-wide numbering systems, or pictograms, you must always keep the understanding and cultural perceptions of users in mind. As a result, you will naturally arrive at consistency and simplicity.

But who are your patients and visitors? The elderly, many with failing vision? Young families with multiple children? What level of education and literacy do they have? Are you a tertiary care center with many out-of-town or international visitors? Does your community see waves of migrant workers at different times of year? Do they speak English? Can they read, in either English or their native language?

And what do you want to provide for these patients and visitors? Say you want to provide bilingual signs in Spanish and English. Excellent, but you consider more than just this superficial ideal. You do not need to provide Spanish signs in the operating room, right? Which dialects will you use? Do you wish to completely accommodate each individual in every situation or to accomplish some lesser measure of accommodation that is less costly? You may choose to provide a personal translator to accompany non-English speakers rather than create every sign, map, and policy in multiple languages; either way, providing communication in a second language is a major commitment, especially if Spanish is not the only foreign language in question.

Furthermore, do only as much as is required by regulatory codes, and you may fall short of your mission to reach out to minority groups. No administrator wants to find himself faced with television cameras and reporters asking, "Why isn't your facility accessible to the Hispanic community?"

Applicable Codes and Standards

There is no lack of horror stories about hospitals failing to comply with little-known or incorrectly applied codes and standards. Consider this example: An inspector directed a facility to install skylights in the operating room because he "felt" it was good to have natural light in that area. When the director of facilities asked for a reference to the code requiring the skylights, the inspector responded, "It is not in any code, and if you press the issue, you will win this battle. However, I can guarantee you will never open this hospital while I am the head inspector."

Do not become one of the organizations that experiences such failures. Be proactive and consult early with inspectors in the region about which codes are being enforced in your area and, more important, how they are being interpreted in the field.

For example, a national life safety standard may call for stairway signs to be mounted on the doors to the stairwells, while the Americans with Disabilities Act (ADA) mandates that the signs are to be posted to the side of the doors. Which do you follow—both? Typically, the more dominant, that is, the most diligently enforced, code dictates position, in this case the ADA. In some cases, you may resort to erecting duplicate signs to satisfy different standards. Your own team may be more knowledgeable about this matter than is the inspector, but this is one example of when to abandon territorial behaviors. You may be technically correct and still find yourself saddled with costly delays. (See chapter 6 for a detailed discussion of codes and standards related to wayfinding.)

Financial Constraints

Just because a hospital across town has addressed its needs in a given manner does not necessarily make it a viable model for your facility. Its resources may be vast compared with yours. Keep in mind that the style you adopt has to fit with the resources—monies and personnel—available going forward for maintenance and updating, as well as for initial sign fabrication and installation. Most signs are purchased in large quantities as one line item; purchasing smaller quantities down the road can cost significantly more. For that matter, even if you can get a replacement at the original unit cost, a single sign may cost hundreds of dollars, an amount that was buried in that first big order.

Start the project in a manner you can afford to continue. For example, a common mistake is to try to make signage elements vandal proof. First, "vandal resistant" may be a more realistic standard. Second, if you blow your entire fabrication budget upfront, how many signs will you be able to afford to clean, repair, or replace every year?

Quality

If "high quality" is the beginning and end of your requirements, it will be hard to tell whether you have succeeded. Therefore, be specific in your requirements, and use concrete language. Do you really need the same imported marble you plan to use for the entrance of the new patient tower in the staff lunchroom as well? Must all the informational brochures in the facility be manufactured in the four-color process? If you have solid core countertops in very prominent spaces or used as accents, can you make do with traditional Plexiglas, at half the price, elsewhere?

Not all parts of the facility are on the "front line" in terms of overall visibility and making a good impression. If you plan to escort patients once they enter a department such as X-ray, then you have the luxury of scaling back signage and using less expensive materials in those areas. You must be able to draw those lines.

Figure 4-2 shows the hierarchy of importance of various areas (or departments) within

Figure 4-2. Hierarchy of Area Importance within Facilities

Keep the main thing, the main thing.

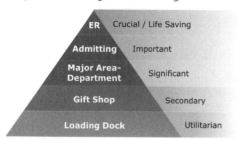

the facility. That hierarchy should drive the priority of the signage for that area. In addition to the volume of traffic and the visibility of the area, consider the importance of that area.

Overall Aesthetic Tone

Signage involves a delicate balancing act as you try to accentuate the natural and built environments without overwhelming them: You want a strong visual presence without being heavy-handed. But what kind of presence?

"Nice" is not a guideline. Do you want the overall effect to be sophisticated? Simple? Colorful? Subdued? Traditional? Contemporary? Abstract? Further, do not assume that everyone understands the relevant terms in the same way. Instead, share pictures that represent the terms' meaning to you.

Keep in mind that the wayfinding program does not exist in isolation: You want it to be in synch with the aesthetic of the facility as a whole; indeed, you want to promote the brand efforts of the organization wherever possible. For example, if your organization is working to implement the Planetree concept, you may want your signage to reinforce that sensibility with wood grains, earth tones, and design elements drawn from nature.

In order to reach agreement on all of these considerations, you must determine the needs for presentation and prototypes. Who needs to review and approve design concepts, and what media will best convey them? Pro-

totypes are a tangible way to test and refine concepts as well as to make sure everyone with a say fully understands what he or she is agreeing to. But sometimes drawings, models, samples, or some combination of these can serve just as well. The key is for the committee to specify what it wants to see—perhaps a PowerPoint presentation, a simple sketch, or a detailed mock-up—and what elements will be required for presentation to the final authority, if this authority does not reside with the committee members.

BUDGETING

There is no quicker way to kill a project than to design it with no one poised to get it funded. A good wayfinding design consultant will be able to tell you how much it will cost to accomplish your goals, but you will need an internal champion to gain commitment from administration and ensure that the money is available when it is needed.

Making the case for investing in an effective wayfinding program should not be difficult once the decision makers grasp the potential return on investment, a measure that can be calculated by what the organization is losing now as a result of *not* having effective wayfinding: expensive staff time.

For example, one large hospital in the Midwest found that 30 percent of first-time visitors and 15 percent of all visitors reported confusion; staff spent an average of 2.4 minutes per encounter to give directions. Even worse, a quarter of those staff asked did not know how to find destinations they were asked about. Twenty-eight percent of staff used "homegrown" wayfinding work-arounds that would not be appropriate for patients and families, such as to allow or escort people through restricted areas. More striking still is what resulted in this hospital when a patient was late for a scheduled appointment: 10.3 percent of the time, staff are idle; 7 percent of the time, equipment is idle; and 31 percent of the time, both equipment and staff are idle.

Figure 4-3 illustrates a project that achieved a return on investment. This urgent care facility's signage featured a large, attractive logo in brushed aluminum when the building first opened to the public. Two years later it replaced the logo fixture with the flag-shaped, internally illuminated urgent care sign shown and saw an immediate 40 percent increase in traffic, making obvious the fact that the more utilitarian sign should have been chosen from the beginning.

Where the money will come from is another issue. Will the plan be paid for out of capital funds, a construction budget, individual department budgets, or the marketing budget? An American Hospital Association wayfinding survey shows that the construction or engineering budget is the most common source of wayfinding funds.[1] This discussion is not meant to dictate how to organize your internal budgeting process. Be advised, though, that when an individual department pays, it tends to feel like it is in charge of the wayfinding process and may refuse to follow a plan that is developed and enforced by another group. Those who are required to pay may resent having no voice in the proposal.

Funds are always finite, so it is also wise to consider breaking the plan into phases so it can be funded accordingly.

Remember that, given the dynamic nature of the health care industry, the cost and ease of updates and changes (including the higher cost for smaller orders of replacement signs mentioned earlier) must be factored into the wayfinding budget from the start.

Cost is basically a simple formula made complex. It involves determining the raw materials needed, the required process to convert them into a finished product, and the built-in profit and overhead amounts.

Estimates may be stated in a variety of ways: as a set amount per door for interior cost estimates (e.g., $150 to $175), as a set amount per bed (e.g., $1,500 per bed for interior and $2,500 per bed for exterior), or as a percentage of the overall new construction budget (e.g., 1 percent to 2 percent of the total). Renovations are much more difficult to estimate until the scope of the project has been determined. In any case, these are at best averages. As the project develops, those in charge will gain experience with new and replacement items. Then the budget can be changed to reflect the new and more accurate estimates of future cost.

Figure 4-3. Sample Signage Demonstrating a Return on Investment

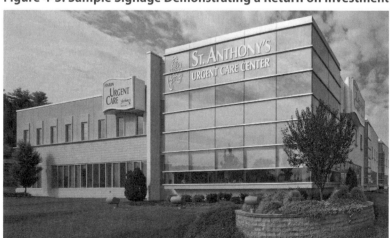

Photo by Debbie Franke Photography.

Following is a list of key factors in determining budget and cost to implement a wayfinding program:

- Scope of the project (i.e., inclusive of signage, kiosks, printed materials like maps, etc.)
- Complexity of the wayfinding needs (those at more complicated facilities cost more to implement)
- Desired aesthetics (usually driven by brand or image criteria)
- Degree of interchangeability
- Choice of completely new system or expansion of existing program
- Available pool of vendor sources and market conditions
- Code compliance

PROJECT TIMELINE

Many comprehensive wayfinding projects can take a year from the time when a problem is first identified to the final implementation. Your signs are not stock items sitting somewhere on a shelf waiting for pickup; they are custom designed and handcrafted to meet the unique needs of your organization. Fabrication and installation are sometimes handled by separate contract, which will need to be put out for bid.

It is natural to want to know how long your project will take. Unfortunately, a timeline is difficult to determine with accuracy, because so many variables depend on how quickly and smoothly the process moves through the bureaucracy of the organization. The design consultant and his team should be able to state without equivocation the length of time steps will take to complete on their end. Once the vendor's time frame is defined, then your organization dictates how the project progresses. At that point, you must decide whether you accept the vendor's offered timeline and plans.

If you need to make changes, now is the time to request them.

But the biggest gaps in the schedule typically occur when your plan hits the desk of someone in the organization for whom it is not a top priority. For example, it is not uncommon to ask someone to review a message schedule that includes literally thousands of individual signs. A message schedule:

- Lists the exact text of every sign, exactly as it is to appear on the finished sign, including capitalization, contractions, punctuation, and abbreviations
- Contains a numeric list of signs whose numbering corresponds to approximate locations on a site plan or floor plan
- Indicates the size and corresponding sign type or format unique to the specific sign
- May indicate construction updates or special notes

Reviewing a message schedule is an overwhelming task and can bog down a project.

Like construction projects, wayfinding can take a design-bid-build approach or can be negotiated as a design-build process. A stripped-down, traditional timeline for the more complicated former approach will look something like that shown in figure 4-4.

The timeline will end with the project's completion, but regular maintenance is ongoing and must be scheduled, and the program's fundamentals must be periodically reviewed after implementation. Many organizations revisit the program 6 to 12 months after it is in place. In addition, someone at the organization should be charged to perform an annual check-up on wayfinding, a task that should be included as a responsibility in her job description and performance review. This check-up should include monitoring complaints and evaluating the impact of new construction whenever it is scheduled.

Figure 4-4. Basic Timeline for a Wayfinding Project: Traditional Approach
The sum of a collective pooling of talent enhances each discipline's efforts.

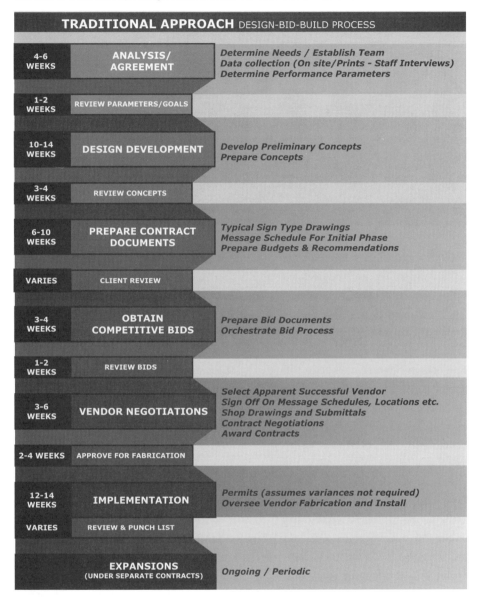

TRADITIONAL APPROACH DESIGN-BID-BUILD PROCESS

4-6 WEEKS	ANALYSIS/ AGREEMENT	*Determine Needs / Establish Team* *Data collection (On site/Prints - Staff Interviews)* *Determine Performance Parameters*
1-2 WEEKS	REVIEW PARAMETERS/GOALS	
10-14 WEEKS	DESIGN DEVELOPMENT	*Develop Preliminary Concepts* *Prepare Concepts*
3-4 WEEKS	REVIEW CONCEPTS	
6-10 WEEKS	PREPARE CONTRACT DOCUMENTS	*Typical Sign Type Drawings* *Message Schedule For Initial Phase* *Prepare Budgets & Recommendations*
VARIES	CLIENT REVIEW	
3-4 WEEKS	OBTAIN COMPETITIVE BIDS	*Prepare Bid Documents* *Orchestrate Bid Process*
1-2 WEEKS	REVIEW BIDS	
3-6 WEEKS	VENDOR NEGOTIATIONS	*Select Apparent Successful Vendor* *Sign Off On Message Schedules, Locations etc.* *Shop Drawings and Submittals* *Contract Negotiations* *Award Contracts*
2-4 WEEKS	APPROVE FOR FABRICATION	
12-14 WEEKS	IMPLEMENTATION	*Permits (assumes variances not required)* *Oversee Vendor Fabrication and Install*
VARIES	REVIEW & PUNCH LIST	
	EXPANSIONS (UNDER SEPARATE CONTRACTS)	*Ongoing / Periodic*

DESIGN DEVELOPMENT

Design development typically involves signage layout and type styles as well as signage construction details. See appendix B for illustrations of these elements. (Lists and specifications of signs to be fabricated and a floor plan showing the location of each sign are developed as part of the documentation and are discussed later in this chapter.)

The Design Team

Design is a collaborative process. Your wayfinding design consultant is responsible for designing your wayfinding program but will most likely bring in other individuals from outside the organization—either from his own firm or from the larger design community—to contribute to the process (figure 4-5). If the latter, the consultant will identify and vet these people and, in

Figure 4-5. Contributors to the Design Process
As with an orchestra, each discipline brings a unique contribution. Under the direction of an experienced wayfinding design consultant, the whole can be bigger and better than the sum of its parts.

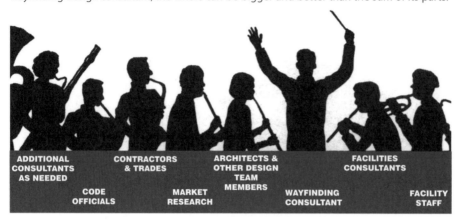

many cases, interview and select them; however, some wayfinding committees prefer to perform these final steps themselves, or at least participate. Indeed, your organization may already have a relationship with one or more design professionals whom you will want to use.

Depending on the nature and scope of your project, the design team may include some or all of the following experts.

An architect. The architect is responsible for conceptualizing the overall project vision and conveying that concept to the rest of the team. In the best-case scenario, this person has been deeply involved with the master planning of the facility or served on the board and has valuable insights into wayfinding needs and opportunities, starting with how the organization's footprint will be changing to accommodate new developments in marketing and technology. If the organization has its own architect on staff, that person would naturally be on the wayfinding committee from the beginning. In any case, it is up to the architect to ensure that the lexicon of signs complements the overall design of the facility.

A general contractor. The general contractor has to make all of various other functions work together. (In many cases, the design consultant will play this role herself.) The contractor will

work closely with the design team to finalize plans for power requirements for all signs that require it, deal with any permit issues, acquire easements, and cope with additional structures (e.g., electrical service boxes, alarm pulls, oxygen lines) that may interfere with the plan.

Subcontractors. What is behind that wall? Will that ceiling support the communication devices we are planning to suspend from it? Subcontractors—brickmasons, electricians, and other workers—will provide valuable information about what can and cannot be done based on conditions that are not readily apparent to the casual observer.

An interior designer. The interior designer understands the physical programming of the facility—how clinical and support programs interact, how traffic flows (and needs to flow)—as well as the aesthetics of the campus. He will suggest how colors and textures can work to promote wayfinding objectives and how space can be created to accommodate wayfinding landmarks.

A landscape architect. Do not think of this person as a glorified groundskeeper but rather as someone who is fluent in the native elements of your site and knows how to create pathways that will see visitors into the buildings naturally and logically. A good landscape architect can create a streetscape that complements the exterior elements of the building or campus and promotes wayfinding.

A Web designer. The last thing you want is a Web site that goes its own way and is inconsistent with signs and handouts in terms of tone, terminology, and information provided. For many people, the site will be their introduction to your facility, and it should prepare for them for what they will find when they actually arrive.

A campus or facilities planner. This person is involved in the development and implementation of the organization's master plan; she may be a full- or part-time employee of the hospital or system or may be hired on a project basis.

First Steps in Design Development

Among the design team's first tasks for design development are to:

- Identify common destinations— laboratories, X-ray, cafeteria, admitting, business office, and so forth—and preferred routes. For example, the shortest route is not always the best if it sends patients through a support services corridor.
- Isolate and study decision points, where a person will need to either change direction or continue along the same path, for visual distractions. Is the lighting adequate? What is the line of sight? Is anything blocking essential information?
- Determine optimal viewing distances and speed. From how far away—and at what speed—should people to be able to read a given sign? A 4-inch letter may be appropriate on a street sign but oversized for inside use.

Figure 4-6. Driver Focus: Basic Factors for Exterior Sign Placement
This figure gives some idea of what it takes to make a sign effective if it is to be seen by a driver.

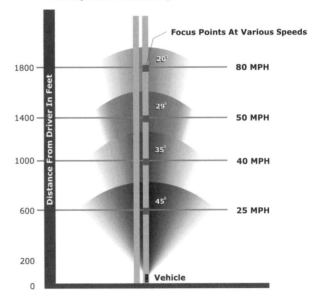

Basic Factors For Exterior Sign Placement

▸ Viewing Distance (See Chart Below)
▸ Code Compliance
▸ Unobstructed 'Line Of Sight'
▸ Avoiding Utilities
▸ Adequate Time To Safely Change Lanes If Needed
▸ Proximity To Entrance (Prior To Drive)
▸ Compensating For Visual Clutter
▸ Terrain (Right Side Of Road Is Preferred)
▸ Providing Power For Illuminated Signs

Design Concepts

This section provides a set of guidelines that all members of the design team should keep in mind. A traditional approach to wayfinding for visitors to health care organizations includes four basic methods:

- *Land ho*: being able to see, recognize, and get to your destination
- *Blinders on*: relying on someone or something—like directional wands and color strips on floors—to escort you
- *Visual cues*: using signs and landmarks as visual cues
- *Mapping*: providing enough information in a printed handout, on a wall fixture, or in some other form to allow people to form a mental map

In most cases, a well-planned program will incorporate some elements of each method, making it effective for the widest range of users.

Most design teams strive to create something new and exciting. This mind-set can be good or bad, depending on whether their innovations are also practical and useful. If so, congratulations are in order; if not, you may have to impose some degree of restraint. One example of lack of restraint is the use of multiple typefaces just because they are available (as is sometimes seen in office newsletters, for example). Certainly there is no need to deliberately shun time-proven methods, and wayfinding may not be the best place to put the organization at risk.

But this caution does not mean you should discourage your design team from proposing wild cards as options to the traditional, emulative, or innovate concepts described earlier in this chapter, as long as there is a sound rationale for them. Not long ago, touch screens were ruled out as a means to gather information because they were considered off-putting and impractical; now they are commonplace at many banks and stores, and they are emerging in the hospital wayfinding function because someone had the audacity to propose them as an option.

Whether time tested or cutting edge, design concepts must take account of the following considerations.

Existing elements. If it isn't broken, don't fix it. For that matter, even if it is broken, you may be able to salvage parts of it. How are people finding their way around now?

Form, function, cost, and durability. Your final selection of materials and techniques should reflect a balance of all four of these elements. If the design comes to exceed the budget, the features should be prioritized and then cheaper alternatives chosen, which is much better done at design time than after implementation.

Flexibility. Most committees want to check flexibility off as a must-have and then move on, but context is key: A wipe-off board with a pen is flexible but not always appropriate—is it meant to convey daily schedules in a conference room, display a menu that changes three times day, or provide patient care information that needs an immediate response?

Some swing-use spaces house different clinics and staff on different days, but to list every activity would take up an entire wall. The solution may be a modular system in which the room number is permanent—raised and in Braille to comply with ADA—and the room description is semipermanent and thus easily changed. Special scrutiny is needed when deciding which and how many individual names are listed on a plaque, sometimes desired solely for reasons of ego.

Planned obsolescence. Although good design is somewhat timeless, colors, basic forms, and other design elements inevitably date a building. Engraved signs with white type on a wood-grain background in a wood frame, for example, may send people into a time warp. Make sure your signage can age gracefully and change with market conditions.

Expandability. Can the wayfinding elements be expanded easily and cost-effectively? Keep in mind that producing small quantities of signs can be more expensive than producing large quantities. Also, think ahead to campus or building additions that are already scheduled for construction. If you are using a facility-wide numbering system, how will such additions be incorporated into that system?

Interaction with other components of the built environment. Unlike some commercial applications, signs for health care facilities should accentuate rather than overpower their surroundings. Although each sign is unique in text and has a distinct purpose, it needs to work with the surroundings as well as with other signs. How will the signage system inter-

Figure 4-7. Sample Signage Demonstrating Planned Obsolescence

This sign incorporates the same faux stucco as is on the building and has changeable panels, making it

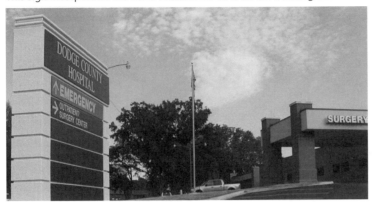

more timeless in appearance: As long as the building is in style, so is the signage. The intention is that the part of the sign that matches the building will be appropriate as long as the building lasts, while the changeable panels will allow for updating to match new fashions.

act with other branding elements, especially those that are meant to make a service line, such as a cancer center or a reproductive health center, stand apart?

Visual hierarchy. All elements of the facility need to be taken into account in the overall plan. For example, new literature racks and magazine tables can either be part of a fight for visual dominance or fit gracefully into the overall scheme, appreciated for their aesthetic contribution but not allowed to interfere with signage or key decision points.

Maintenance. You may love the look of that imported marble, but what will it demand in terms of time, materials, and expense to keep it looking beautiful? Perhaps begin by asking your cleaning and maintenance crews, or even outsiders, what long-term upkeep requires.

Size versus impact. Size does matter—but so do placement, contrast, glare, competing elements, and preconceptions. Just because one can read the last line on the eye chart while focusing under controlled lighting in the optometrist's office does not mean the person can read 3-inch lettering on a street sign as he dashes by at night. Also, just because a message is legible does not mean it achieves the desired effect. Review the information provided earlier for the factors that the design team must attend to in order to ensure that a sign is effective.

DESIGNING GREEN: DOING MORE WITH LESS

"Green" is a mind-set, a commitment—and, increasingly, a sound business approach. As our planet melts, green (or sustainable) building is on its way to becoming a given method of construction. Wayfinding typically is only a small part of the building process, albeit a highly visible one, but graphic designers nevertheless have a contribution to make in terms of their effect on the environment.

The Society for Environmental Graphic Design has identified the following five strategies for incorporating sustainability into graphic design projects, all built around the theme of longevity, or performance over time:

- Air and environmental quality—select products and procedures that contain reduced levels of volatile organic compounds (VOCs), which emit pollutants into the air
- Resource and waste management
- End-of-usable-life management—for example, recycling
- Energy and lighting efficiency
- Education and interpretation—informing the public of green aspects of the project

Choosing to use green products and fabrication processes—including material selection and final disposition as products reach the end of their life cycle—will keep your wayfinding program from adding to the already large carbon footprint most hospitals represent. Neither designers nor clients want to sacrifice graphic quality or aesthetic value for sustainability, and there is no need to do so. Ask your designer or consultant about her experience in this area.

For example, you can exert environmental leadership by making sure your signage and other wayfinding elements incorporate the following whenever possible:

- Low-pressure, high-volume, water-based paint systems
- Low-VOC paints and sealants
- Modular products with paper or other recyclable inserts that allow signs to remain undisturbed while being updated
- Energy-efficient lighting in light-emitting diode (LED) systems and solar power sources
- Screws instead of glues for assembly and mounting

These steps represent significant design decisions, and although you may well be able to achieve both, utility trumps beauty every time. Match the background of a sign to the wallpaper beneath it, and you may have achieved a beautiful area that people walk right by without noticing. One off-campus clinic, illustrated earlier in this chapter in figure 4-3, found that its large brushed aluminum logo on reflective glass was aesthetically pleasing, but

when it was replaced by a much smaller and plainer but more obvious and descriptive new sign, patient traffic doubled within a week.

TYPOGRAPHY: WHEN "BIGGER" ISN'T ALWAYS "BETTER"

Eye charts demonstrate that a 1-inch letter can be read by the average viewer from approximately 25 feet away. But take a look at the two letters below. Both are simple letter forms in 72-point type, but are they equally readable?

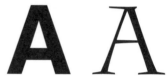

Figure 4-8 offers an illustration of simple readability versus visual weighting in two competing layouts. Which is more effective for a visitor's wayfinding?

Another issue related to impact and readability is that of letter height. The assumption is that as you double the height of a letter, you double its visual mass. In fact, you are also doubling the width, yielding four times the visual impact.

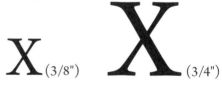

X (3/8")   X (3/4")

Figure 4-9 offers a viewing distance guide for sign placement. The guide provides rec-

Figure 4-8. Sample Signage Demonstrating Visual Weighting

The layout on the left is functional but not attractive. The layout on the right emphasizes the firm name and the suite number, which is what patients are looking for.

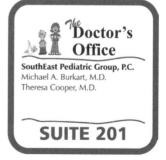

201

The Doctor's Office
Southeast Pediatric Group, P.C.
Michael A. Burkart, M.D.
Theresa Cooper, M.D.

The Doctor's Office

SouthEast Pediatric Group, P.C.
Michael A. Burkart, M.D.
Theresa Cooper, M.D.

SUITE 201

ommendations for various letter heights to achieve the maximum desired viewing distances.

Once the signage system has been designed, you will need to establish criteria and a process for updating and adding to it before you enjoy your accomplishment. Who can request a new sign? Who is authorized for approval? How quickly can decisions be made and executed? These questions will be easier to answer if you have documentation, as discussed in the next section.

PREPARING DOCUMENTATION

The deliverables of the wayfinding project include, among other elements, control documents that summarize findings and decisions and describe what is being purchased in terms of analysis, design, and implementation. This documentation is known as *disbursement*, an architecture term referring to a set of drawings and specifications and a description of the tangible items expected to be delivered related to the design contract.

Figure 4-9. Viewing Distance Guide

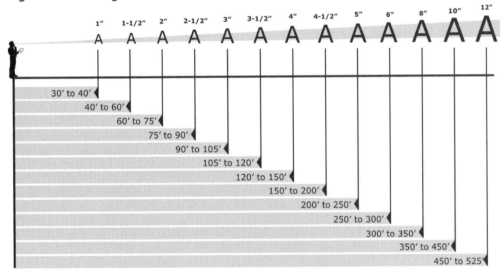

GUIDE FOR *MAXIMUM* VIEWING DISTANCES

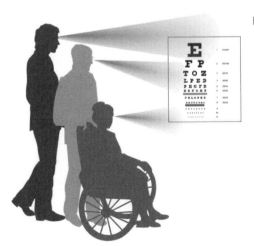

LETTER SIZING

Letter size is dependent upon a number of factors as noted:

▸ Viewers eyesight.

▸ Angle of acuity without turning or tilting the head.

▸ Viewing distance & desired visual impact.

▸ Letter contrast with background color and glare

▸ Lighting conditions in the area in which the sign is to be located.

▸ Clear line of sight.

▸ Simple letterform.

▸ Minimal visual clutter to compete with.

You should require the following control documents from your design consultant:

- A report of the on-site survey
- Conceptual review models
- A signage system manual (including a section on policy and procedures)

Report of the On-Site Survey

This report should have been submitted at the end of the needs analysis and prior to the preliminary design phases, and it should have served to bring every committee member into alignment on the project's scope (see chapter 3). The report should include an evaluation of existing conditions; a list of measurable goals, with targets, for committee consideration; a list of performance criteria or parameters, also for committee consideration; a list of primary destinations; a map or description of desired pathways; and a list or map of key decision points. Also included should be an overview of applicable codes and standards. This document becomes the foundation for a determination of parameters and project performance criteria by the wayfinding committee.

Conceptual Review Models

These models are submitted for review and revision after the preliminary design phase but before the finalized plan is submitted for approval to the board or executive committee. The review models consist of on-site photos with overlay of potential solutions; detailed, individual drawings of each sign type; illustrated lexicon, showing the complete range of sign types and specifying their size in relation to each other ("This is a family photo, while the previous item is a collection of individual portraits"); prototypes of viable alternatives, such as representative sign types, including materials, colors, and textures; and budget options based on various design scenarios. Photos of similar products at other facilities

will help decision makers visualize the final product once it is fully implemented.

Signage System Manual

This manual is submitted before the implementation phase (see chapter 5). It includes basic control drawings (with backup disk) indicating, for each sign type, the construction details, materials, size, colors, formats, and layouts; a list of typical terminology; a completion schedule; a floor plan indicating all sign locations; control samples of colors and finishes; and reorder documents.

Policy and Procedures

One section of the signage system manual—policy and procedures—is submitted toward the end of the project, before (and to be used in) staff training. The policy and procedures section includes the name and contact information of the in-house signage coordinator; an approved vendor list for outsourced items and as backup material; procedure forms for requesting a new or updated sign and replacing an outdated or damaged sign; established routes to common destinations; correct terminology for locations; a schedule for periodic reassessment of needs and the program as a whole; forms for logging requests for directions and complaints; target measures used to gauge the success of the program; and a maintenance schedule.

A CLOSER LOOK AT THE SIGNAGE SYSTEM MANUAL

This manual is the bible of your signage system; you will use it to construct as well as maintain the system, so the long-term health of the wayfinding program is based on the quality of this document. Even people who are yet to be hired into the organization will need to depend on this document in the future to show them how to carry on the work you have planned, so it must be very clear, leaving no factors to chance.

Following is a list of typical elements that should be included in the manual:

- Illustrated lexicon: interior and exterior.
- Details of any concept intent, such as color-coded quadrants.
- Construction details indicating materials and techniques.
- Typography, illustrated and with arrows.
- Installation and mounting placement criteria.
- Typical layout of each sign by type (a categorization by function).
- Indication for the use of each sign type. For example, can a sign reading "Environmental Services" be used for a basic room identification plaque or for larger department identification signage? Depending on where the sign is located, it could be used for either: On the floors, multiple environmental services department signs (e.g., "Broom Closet") will be needed, while only one door will serve as the entrance to the environmental services department, which requires a larger sign.
- Specifications of construction details, materials, and performance criteria.
- Schedule of messages for every sign in the project.
- Sign location plan that corresponds to the message schedule.
- Unit pricing and extended prices.
- Information needed to reorder and update every sign type and module.
- Documentation of collateral materials, such as electronic and print materials, and how they integrate with the overall wayfinding program.

Signs are grouped by similarity in function. For example, a D-1 type sign might indicate a primary directional module, while an RR-2 type sign might indicate a staff-only washroom. It is not enough to have someone show you a sketch and say, "This type of sign will look like this, only it will be bigger and blue instead of red." You need to see full-size prototypes of each.

As you might imagine, the floor plan cannot show the actual signs, which might number in the hundreds or thousands. Instead, numbers are used that refer to a document spelling out what each sign actually says. So, for example, sign 47 reads "Chief Nursing Officer," with Mary Smith as an insert.

Details such as specifications, construction techniques, and layouts are all part of the sign systems documentation (see figures 4-10 and 4-11 for examples). Collectively, they are referred to as the "contract documents," and they become the legal foundation should a dispute occur in the fabrication process. For example, specifications can indicate company A's Series XYZ product, or they can indicate those materials or construction techniques that are acceptable. Specifications can also indicate

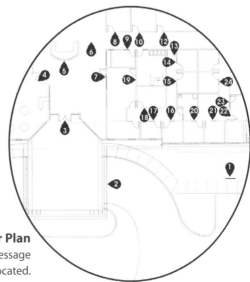

Figure 4-10. Sample Architectural Floor Plan
Architectural floor or site plans with corresponding message schedules document where each sign is to be located.

Figure 4-11. Sample Shop Drawings

While the drawing on the left is adequate to convey design intent, shop drawings like that on the right show construction details.

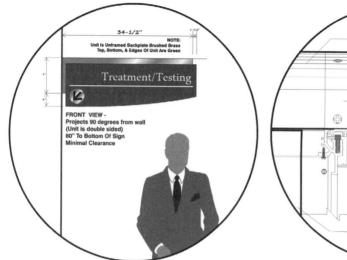

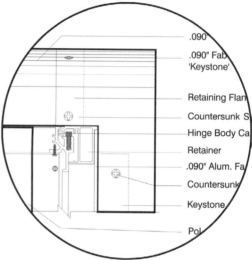

what tolerances are acceptable or what products or techniques are not acceptable.

Articulating details such as these can be a daunting task and usually includes some broad clauses such as, "Field verify all locations/conditions/final messages." In preparing the documents for the manual, care must be taken to limit the design team's liability through insurance and clauses on the "adequacy and accuracy of information provided" in the specifications to throw much of the burden back to the fabricator.

Tongue in cheek, it is said that "If the designer makes a mistake, it is the sign guy's fault." The simple truth is that the designer designs and the fabricator builds to the design intent.

Tools that the designer provides to the fabricator to ensure that the fabricator receives the necessary and expected information are called *submittals* and include the following:

- Shop drawings showing in great detail how the products are made
- A prototype of specific typical sign elements

- Actual color samples
- Proofs of printed materials
- A preview of electronic media prior to going live

Submittals should be viewed with a critical eye and not accepted with comments such as, "The final product will be like this, only better." If anything, the opposite is usually true.

The manual also needs to address the possibility that the sign supplier might go out of business or that your relationship with it might deteriorate. What backup provisions have been formulated? Who maintains the ownership or creative rights to the artwork generated?

Once your wayfinding project is budgeted, designed, and documented, you are ready to move on to the next phase: implementation.

REFERENCE

1. Cooper Signage & Graphics for Society for Healthcare Strategy and Market Development (SHSMD) and AHA Solutions, "Wayfinding Needs of Health Care Facilities." Needs Determination Series. Chicago: SHSMD and AHA Solutions, 2008.

CHAPTER 5

Implementation

I mplementation is never an overnight process, certainly not in today's economic environment. Instead, it usually takes place in several stages, based on construction requirements, political realities, budgets, and other priorities.

The typical stages include the following:

1. Production—fabrication and installation of signs
2. Rollout and phasing, including prototyping and beta field testing
3. Staff training
4. Additional phasing, as needed
5. Periodic review and updating—at least annually

All five stages are aspects of good project management. Another factor in successful project management is avoiding common pitfalls. The following list examines these pitfalls before addressing the stages.

- Not adhering to the schedule
  For example: getting bogged down in the review process, not setting up subcommittees if and when needed to handle the workflow, failing to follow priorities, capitulating to "scope creep"
- Failing to commit sufficiently to the project
  For example: not gaining buy-in from the top down at each stage of the project, underbudgeting, not assigning or enforcing accountability
- Undermining program standards
  For example: making random exceptions to established guidelines, allowing privileged groups to insist on a separate set of standards, slacking off on enforcement
- Not establishing a central authority to update and maintain the program
  For example: splitting the job among several people, allowing the sign maker to decide what size or kind of sign is appropriate, expecting individual departments to conduct periodic needs assessment
- Using old processes but expecting new results
  For example: insisting on bidding a project when past experience at your organization suggests that the process often means involving a series of vendors over multiple project phases, thus sacrificing continuity, quality, and relationships; buying from catalogs because the products featured in them are cheap but expecting a higher quality level or better service than that vendor has provided in the past; buying local to support the community even if the local vendor

> Design is not just what it looks like. Design is how it works. Steve Jobs

pool is limited in health care work; buying the lowest-priced product and expecting it to be equal in quality to more expensive products

- Trying to fit the project into a mold developed for another project
  For example: allowing the fabricator to order materials based on "catalog sizes" instead of customized specifications, failing to cut blanket purchase orders, not acknowledging receipt of signage materials that bypass the loading dock

Keep these pitfalls in mind as you prepare for each stage of implementation.

FABRICATION: DESIGN-BID-BUILD VERSUS DESIGN-BUILD

There is more than one way to complete the job of fabricating and installing signs. Stated simply, design-bid-build (D-B-B) is the tradi-

tional method for project delivery, in which the designer and her team prepare the tender documents on which general contractors bid; the contractor who is awarded the contract fabricates and installs the signs, with or without the help of subcontractors. Design-build (D-B) is a streamlined process in which a single entity (the designer-builder, designer–sign broker, or design-build contractor) handles the design as well as the fabrication and installation; this method is comparable to fast-track scenarios in construction in that the firm selected to implement the program from start to finish is held accountable for all results, including adherence to a predetermined budget.

Each method carries advantages and disadvantages. Obviously, D-B is faster—the documentation and submittal process will take two to three months less time—and, for that reason, often more cost-effective (see figure 5-1). Accountability is straightforward with a single

Figure 5-1. Basic Timeline for a Wayfinding Project: Solutions Approach

Taking a design-build approach can save significant time and money as well as streamline communications, but only if you are comfortable with the relationship.

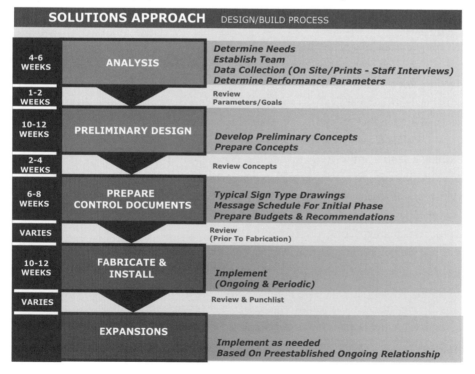

doc
loca
- *Is th*
  sam
  you
  reas
- *Say*
  sign
  com
- *In w*
  to th
  com
- *Wh*
  sign
  incl
  pole
- *Doe*
  acco
  dizii
- *Wh*
  site,
  For
  shop
  This
  dire
  Som
  only
  non
  side
  to-w
  your
  worl
  ensu
  trad
- *Are*
  or pi
  Usin
  into
  whic
  or in
  orga
  plac
  of ta
  To u

source, and the organization must deal with just one entity for the project: Regardless of how many subcontractors he may use, the designer-builder handles all design revisions, permitting, construction issues, change orders, and billing.

The issue of errors and omissions by the designer-builder is eliminated because he is the fabricator. He accepts the responsibility, which reduces finger-pointing between parties when intention does not match implementation. The D-B method allows you to define the scope and budgets of the project earlier in the project, leaving less room for misunderstandings that often arise during the bidding process (but may not come to light until later) and considerably more room for flexibility, as alterations need not be negotiated and subjected to rebidding.

Some D-B vendors offer rebates on or apply a portion of design fees toward implementation—a savings that should be reflected in the project. This savings can be cycled back into the facility or applied to building prototypes or beta testing, using full-size signs, before committing to a finished product. (No sketch or mock-up can do justice to full-size, in-place signs that can be viewed in a real-world environment and adjusted quickly and with little expense to the entire system. See the "Rollout and Phasing" section later in this chapter for more discussion on beta testing.)

The design-build process tends to be much less document- and submittal-intensive—resulting in additional cost savings—but achieving success with this model relies heavily on the quality of the vendor and the vendor-customer relationship. Finally, concern is reduced about your vendors disappearing when the time comes to service your replacement needs. The vendor in a design-build project aims to develop an ongoing, mutually beneficial relationship and has a vested interest in maintaining the integrity of a program. The program is a reference the vendor can draw

upon in discussions with other potential customers. Conversely, an independent designer may have concerns about the availability of long-term maintenance and replacement by the vendor, so she initiates new contracts for each project, even if it is simply a straightforward expansion of the existing lexicon, so the risk is not so great.

The D-B approach requires you to include in the contract all projects that need completing, including master planning for growth whenever possible, because design fees will accrue with each new project or change in scope. Also consider using an initial-bid process to select and cement your vendor relationship for future phases and reorders, as they can be substantial.

On the other hand, as a theoretically impartial third party, the designer in D-B-B can mediate disputes between you and the contractor and will look out for your interests throughout the implementation process, which can also save you time and aggravation. Thanks to the bidding process itself, incomplete, incorrect, or missed items are usually discovered and addressed before fabrication begins, and you are less likely to pay more than is necessary to purchase the products you want. Design fees can be offset by lower bid prices. If you use the D-B-B process, you can—and should—always insert a clause in the bid documents that specifies replacement costs for a specific period, typically a year. Still, a D-B-B project tends to be executed using a more traditional process, and you will need to budget ample time, typically 12 to 24 months, for implementation.

Based on extensive experience, many professionals favor the D-B approach, but ask around, and you will hear strong opinions advocating both methods. The key is to not automatically commit yourself to selecting a company using the same method the organization has always used simply because it has

always
define
expect

In
commi
cons c
which
project
both p
is mos
everyo
stands
the fal
simple
the wc
thousa
("beca
incurri

Prequ

Most c
ries of
accept
bidder,
was nc
priced
sive ch
makes
after bi

To
ships v
ally be
If this
docum
to ach
tion. U
appenc
whose
of thei
Remen
signage
dealers
and do
to exec

modified standard products whenever possible, as innovation carries its own risk. Determine in advance how the vendor defines the term *or equal* when used as a qualifier for a specific product. Negotiate reorder prices upfront; the process and implications of carving out money from a large capital budget are much different from doing so for ongoing budget line items.

It is important that much detail be included in the bid documents, but keep in mind that designers will charge more to include more detail. Avoid seeking an unreasonable amount of detail in the documents. On the other hand, be sure to examine the bids closely. If, for example, you specify aluminum for exterior signs but fail to indicate the thickness, you are inviting bidders to use their own judgment, and each may assess the need differently. The low bidder may plan to use much thinner aluminum than you had in mind.

In addition, when using the traditional design-bid-build method, you must be sure to purchase errors and omissions insurance for the design firm, if it does not have its own policy in place. If the firm fails to fulfill a significant portion of the project, neither you nor the contractor will be required to pay the price for its omission.

Finally, because no one can anticipate every eventuality—and the longer you spend on refining the documents in an effort to do so, the more money you spend before you have a single sign in place—make sure language is included in the contract that conveys, in essence, "Mr. Fabricator, if we made a mistake, it's your fault." Too often, hospitals adopt standard language drawn up by the designer that says, for example, "Sign contractor to field verify all conditions and message schedules prior to fabrication and must submit detailed shop drawings and prototypes as requested prior to beginning any work. The designer is not responsible for any errors and omissions."

This language places the onus of satisfactory results on the fabricator, even for cases in which the fabricator may not be at fault for a mistake.

Modular Systems: A Good Value

In the same way that you can either order a custom-tailored suit or buy one off the rack, you can either have your signs designed specially for you or buy standard modular signs that provide good value for a low price; you may also choose to use a combination of the two options. Talk with your design consultant about modular systems to determine if they are a viable option for your signage program.

For both interiors and exteriors, a modular system with a few basic interchangeable components—be they window signs with slide-in inserts produced with desktop publishing, vinyl die cuts on thin card stock, or attachable plaques—gives a permanent appearance to the signage and still allows you to comply with changing accessibility standards and codes. Using standard "off the rack" components has its place; you do not always need to reinvent the wheel when good, field-tested products are appropriate for some needs.

Figures 5-2 and 5-3 show examples of modular systems. You can order standard products from vendors accessible on the Internet, by catalog, or from samples. Depending on your needs, such systems can be suitable in many circumstances and even serve as a valuable part of your wayfinding program. Such signs may be available wholesale to the sign trade or sold through a more restrictive manufacturer's program or some kind of dealer network.

The polar opposite of standard modular systems are custom-designed products. These sign systems can differentiate your organization from other facilities and create a strong impression (figure 5-4). But beware

Figure 5-2. Sample Exterior Modular Signage

Aluminum modular post and panel systems often are the workhorse of many exterior signing systems.

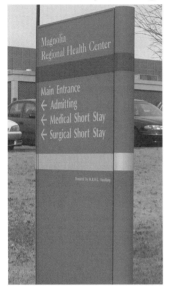

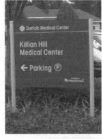

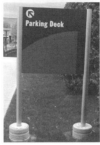

Figure 5-3. Sample Interior Modular Signage

For interior signage, popular modular plaque systems can often fit your needs.

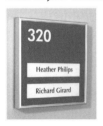

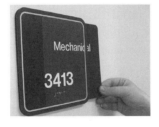

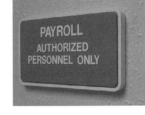

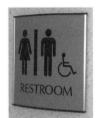

Figure 5-4. Sample Custom-Designed Signage

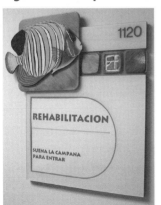

There are times when custom solutions are called for, if for no other reason than to personalize your facility.

the following pitfalls of such "unproven" products:

- They can look great in concept but simply fall short in a real-world environment.
- They can carry some risk if the construction techniques used to create a unique appearance are experimental rather than established.
- They may be expensive or hard to update or replace in small quantities.

To determine whether a modular product is suited to your wayfinding program, the project team should work with the designer and/or contractor to evaluate it against the core project criteria. Can it easily be incorporated into your signage system without compromise? If so, then there is no need to duplicate effort by choosing a completely custom-designed product. If not, do not try to adapt modular products beyond their intended purpose; a custom solution may be more appropriate.

ROLLOUT AND PHASING

Even the best design can be refined economically, or value engineered, as it begins to unfold. Using a small project as a beta test is an appropriate approach, though it is not always possible. In any event, phasing should be determined early, based on the project's goals, schedule, and funding.

One organization constructing a replacement facility avoided later trouble by using an existing building, which was to remain in use, as a beta test for the new signage system. A logo color for the facility was selected based on a new logo for the facility's business cards. The color was an attractive copper in the printed materials. But when the same color was used on the exterior of the building, under different lighting and depending on the time of day, it could appear copper, orange, or salmon. An adjustment to the color was made prior to the completion of the replacement facility. What could have been an expensive and embarrassing problem for the new facility was averted in the test phase of the project.

Retrofitting an existing facility might proceed as outlined in the following list:

Initial phase. Beta test specific areas before implementing the full program: Install prototypes in an enhanced entrance, a small freestanding clinic, or another small area.

Second phase. Interiors: Implement the directional program for the main level and upgrade signage for most public spaces on the main level, especially major areas or departments. Exteriors: Upgrade site identification.

Third phase. Interiors: Implement directional signage for patient room floors; identify public elevators.

Fourth phase. Exteriors: Install secondary identification signs, directional signs, and regulatory signs.

Fifth phase. Address remaining areas as needed.

STAFF TRAINING: THE ART OF GIVING DIRECTIONS

The following is a true story: A well-meaning nurse told a visiting couple looking for the cafeteria that they could "take that elevator right there down to the second floor." Indeed, that was the closest elevator and would open up right outside the cafeteria, and visitors use it all the time. Technically, however, it was designated for staff use only; the waiting couple was greeted by funeral home staff transporting a recently deceased patient to the funeral home. Rather than blame any particular party, one might attribute this unpleasant occurrence to a failure of the wayfinding system: The elevator was not clearly marked and staff had come to think of it simply as the most direct route to the cafeteria. This sort of "homegrown" directing is based on good intentions, but it is not helpful or appropriate.

Giving directions effectively and appropriately in a hospital is something of an art, and training staff how to do it is an important part of the wayfinding program. Training should include not only new staff, who can be educated during basic orientation, but also those staff who have long tenure with the organization and have the more difficult job of unlearning historic nomenclature and bad habits.

Figure 5-5 illustrates the trouble a staff member can cause by giving a visitor poor directions. Good directions follow six key rules:

1. Do not assume the seeker has any knowledge about the facility (unless you know for a fact that he is already operating on faulty or outdated information).
2. Do not give directions as if you, the staff person, were going to the destination; keep shortcuts to and for yourself and your colleagues.
3. Never send visitors through staff-only areas or areas that do not project the image the organization is promoting.
4. Keep it simple: "Take the elevators up ahead on the right to the third floor, then

look for signs when you get off; your destination will be to the right."

5. When helping people on the telephone or off-site, always give directions to the specific entrance and/or parking area appropriate to their destination. As figure 5-6 illustrates, it is not advisable to ask the visitor to rely on architectural cues.

6. If the destination is hard to find, escort the visitor (or find someone else to do so) or arrange for someone to meet him along the way.

There is no special need to separate executive from line staff for the purpose of training; with the exception of volunteers, who should be trained separately, people may be grouped in whatever combinations are convenient and customary. Incorporate role-playing and/or filmed examples of good and bad direction giving, including some unfortunate results of the latter.

In addition to direction giving, in-service training in wayfinding should cover the following topics:

- The rationale for the wayfinding program, including the problems it is designed to solve and the benefits it will deliver to staff as individuals as well as to the organization as a whole.

- The importance of sticking to the rules, such as not putting up paper signs except in an emergency; routing requests for new signs to the proper person; and, when in doubt, checking with the policy and procedures manual for the rules of the program, which should be widely available.

**Figure 5-5. Sample Visitor Pathways:
The "Shortest" versus the "Preferred" Way to a Destination**

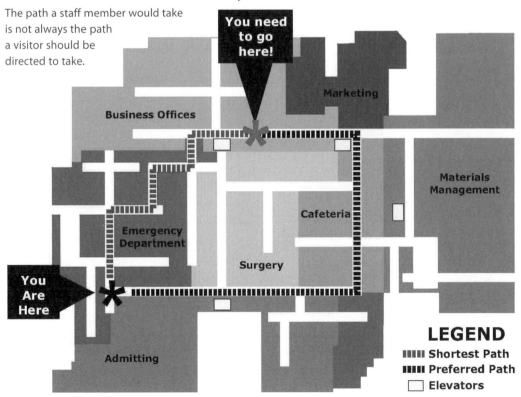

The path a staff member would take is not always the path a visitor should be directed to take.

You need to go here!

Marketing

Business Offices

Materials Management

Cafeteria

Emergency Department

Surgery

You Are Here

Admitting

LEGEND
▦ Shortest Path
▦ Preferred Path
▢ Elevators

Figure 5-6. The Problem with Architectural Cues

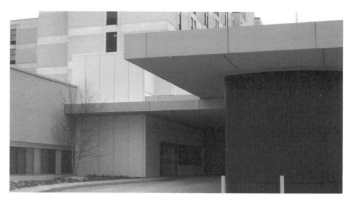

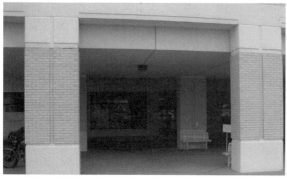

Which of these two entrances to a 900-bed hospital is a public entrance? The one shown on the bottom left is an outpatient entrance, while the one shown on the top right is meant for ambulances only. Do not rely on architectural cues when giving visitors directions.

- The terminology that has been established for the program, including the proper names for wings, entrances, units, departments, and so forth. Make sure all staff have easy access to a clear, well-ordered list of the correct terms.
- The established routes for common destinations—and the need to gradually introduce frequent users of the facility, such as clergy, among visitors and patients to the new paths as appropriate.
- The need to log requests for directions. Develop and provide staff with a standard form and procedure for this purpose, and collect and analyze the data.

Keep in mind that, if the area that has always been called 3-East is now to be know as the Bob Hope Wing, simply saying so once will not encourage staff to eliminate their use of the term *3-East*. Periodic testing on the new terminology and routes will help institutionalize the change, as will making them easy and fun to learn. For example, hold a contest for the first month of the introduction of the new terminology whereby "strangers" randomly ask staff for directions. Those who provide correct directions are rewarded with a small token, such as a $1-off coupon for a purchase in the cafeteria.

PERIODIC REVIEW AND UPDATING

Beyond any additional phasing that may be necessary is a need for periodic review and updating. An effective sign system resembles a business plan in that activity is often intensive in the planning process and initial phases but soon becomes standard operating procedure. But just as with business plans, it is important to revisit the original signage plan from time to time in order to keep it fresh and relevant. Pull the plan out of the drawer and re-evaluate it to consider new developments, including new market strategies, new technology, and new styles; to alter course if and where necessary; and to bring new resources to bear in terms of both personnel and funding.

Often this review can be conducted in-house; occasionally, you may benefit from bringing in an independent expert to provide a more objective review and new ideas.

Obviously, such a review can be triggered by construction or renovation. In addition to these times, establish and adhere to a set schedule (at least annually) of review dates in the absence of other events. In the interim, the person responsible for making weekly maintenance rounds should take notes or snap pictures of signs that need attention.

The high cost of a comprehensive way-finding program may be hidden in a large construction project, but not so with the cost to maintain or update it, which is also significant. A seemingly straightforward decision to move the admissions department to another area, for example, can incur thousands of dollars of cost in directional updates.

One way to keep updating costs under control is to invest in a system that utilizes relatively inexpensive inserts that can be relocated or replaced as needed within more expensive frames and fixtures. This approach is not only cost-effective but also ecologically friendly, because reusing components and updating only as needed are more environmentally friendly practices than producing a new sign and throwing the old one away.

Do It Yourself: The In-House Sign Shop

It may occur to you at this point that you could save considerable money—and improve responsiveness to the need for updating—by making your own signs. Perhaps this idea is valid. Keep in mind, however, that how well or poorly you execute your signage system can translate directly into higher or lower patient satisfaction as well as feed an image that inspires or discourages the market. It is strongly recommended that you avoid manufacturing signs in-house unless you are prepared to do it right: Provide adequate resources; train fabricating staff; buy equipment; designate space; and, most of all, be willing to cease the in-house production operation if its demands are beyond the organization's capabilities and resources.

If you are interested in bringing sign fabrication in-house, give yourself an edge by using a step-by-step approach. First, before making any signs, be sure you have in place a master plan for the entire signage system that aligns with the organization's own master facility plan. This is a good activity in which to invest in some outside expertise. By establishing a master signage plan, you can avoid wasting costly materials, confusing people, and having to backtrack later. It is important to identify and plan for various types of change, from menu items in the cafeteria and patient names on room doors to future plans for expansion of programs and facilities. Modular design, in which a portion of the sign can easily be removed and updated via slide-in panels or changeable post-and-panel systems, is the key to staying current with much of the signage.

Second, select and educate the project team that will oversee or arrange for fabrication, installation, and maintenance of the system. Be sure it gathers input from all areas; each department will have its own ideas about the function and location of signs. Well before implementing the system, the team will need to educate all hospital staff in the importance of having all signs work together as independent yet interrelated elements in a shared environment, and enlist their cooperation.

Third, create consistent and concise terminology that is understandable to the general public as well as to staff. In general, address the lowest common denominator in determining level of communication, that is, the first-time visitor who has relatively poor comprehension skills and is under stress. Keep in mind that even the best of us can read just five to seven words at a time easily; you must translate memos, policies, and other communications into clear, bite-size messages for your visitors.

In one facility, a recent sign request asked for the following text to appear on a sign: "Effective July 1, 2009, this is a healthcare facility and we are concerned for the well-being of the staff, visitors and patients that we serve. Please refrain from the use of tobacco products of any kind. Thank you for not smoking and your help in making this a healing place." What the facility actually needed was a sign that read, "This Is a Tobacco-Free Facility" and a large pictogram. Again, less is often more in communicating messages.

Fourth, make sure you have created a sign system manual, as described in chapter 4, that identifies each type of sign you need—and think you might need in the future—by size, function, color, and construction. Making a sign and designing a sign require two very different sets of skills; it is unlikely that you have the latter skill available in-house. At the very least, you should contract with a graphic artist to establish the design standards.

Fifth, research your options and find out which approaches have worked in organizations similar to your own. For example, the feedback is still mixed on the wisdom of using advanced technology such as talking door signs and touch screen directories in an in-house sign program; they may still experience operational issues and can easily eat up your entire wayfinding program budget.

Sixth, determine what equipment (hardware and software), space, training, time, and consumable items you will need to execute the sign fabrication operation. Typically, the cost of implementation will need to be applied over several budget years.

Finally, start the fabrication operation by performing sign repair, relocation, and installation, and only gradually move into fabricating signs—first for the most frequent and compelling needs of the facility and then eventually for the whole spectrum of needs. Equipment and employees can be added as needs, expertise, and budgets allow.

No matter how you choose to update your wayfinding program, it is important to recognize that wayfinding is a substantial investment and needs updating from time to time. The administration and department heads must be unified in their efforts to maintain its integrity. Paper signs should never be allowed, except in an emergency—and even then, they should be in use for no more than 24 hours.

Equipment Options for In-House Sign Shops

The following sign-making tools and techniques can all be used appropriately in a hospital sign shop.

Vinyl die cuts. These are the most widely used sign-making tools today, helpful for interior signage and essential for exterior signage. They are basically one-color plotters—a kind of large-format printer used by contractors and architects to produce line drawings like floor plans and other prints—with a knife blade substituting for a pen. A four-step process must take place before applying the lettering to a background, using either dedicated input and output devices or an output device for the existing computer system. The four-step process involves the following:

1. Programming the text on specialized sign software
2. Cutting the vinyl material
3. Removing the excess material that does not create the image or lettering
4. Providing a masking film to act as a carrier to maintain special relationships while the vinyl is applied to the substrate

Vinyl has evolved as the standard for non-illuminated lettering on exterior signage. While surface-applied, vinyl-cut letters in various grades are readily available, you may want to set up your own fabricating shop if you plan to use them extensively. The final product is professional, durable, and flexible, but not tactile. Good floodlight fixtures can light the sign and the scene simultaneously.

Desktop publishing. Interior signage can be designed to accept a laser- or inkjet-printed insert (figure 5-7). This process produces an economical sign with minimal equipment and training. Incorporating preprinted color accents or logos often increases the visual integrity of the process. These inserts are not tactile but can be used for semipermanent room identification and directional strips in most states. The U.S. Department of Justice considers them to be reasonable accommodation, understanding that "Community Relations" today might be "Marketing" next week, while the room number, the permanent room identification, will remain "room 1134." Most facilities can upgrade software and output devices for this purpose with little cost and

produce a professional sign insert that satisfies both facility and regulatory requirements.

Engraving. Using the method of engraving to make interior signs was standard for a many years but fell in popularity as more attractive options became available. However, today's engraving methods can produce signs that are more aesthetically pleasing and functional than in the past.

Individually applied letters and Braille. Individually cut or injection-molded letters can be aligned to form words and numbers that are tactile and, in limited use, can be a cost-effective way to provide signage for the visually impaired. (See the plaque on the left in figure 5-8.) Providing a sign system of thousands of individual characters, however, can boggle the mind—and boost the budget. A good rule of thumb is to use applied letters when a specific population needs it or in limited fashion, such as raised numbers in conjunction with semipermanent plaques or inserts.

Photopolymer. This material involves a dedicated, multiple-step process to produce signage graphics. It requires special equipment, skilled labor, and supplies. Nevertheless, the

Figure 5-7. Sample Permanent Frame with Paper Insert

Even Americans with Disabilities Act (ADA)–compliant signs can feature a paper insert with the semipermanent text on the insert and the permanent portion (room number) in raised letters and Braille.

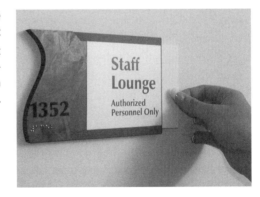

Figure 5-8. Sample Signage for the Visually Impaired

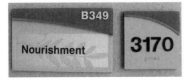

The plaque on the left uses laser/engraver-cut letters bonded to the background material, with individual "rastors" (plastic beads) embedded into the background. The plaque on the right is a one-piece photopolymer with the text tipped, or silk-screened, to render a color that contrasts with the spray-painted background. Both samples represent common methods of fabricating ADA-compliant plaques.

photopolymer technique is the most common method in use by sign professionals for producing high-quality, tactile signs. The result is a monolithic plaque with the background painted and then overlaid with what the industry calls "tipped" copy. (See the plaque on the right in figure 5-8.) The addition of color to the front of the text area is normally silk-screened as a last step in production.

The advantage of photopolymer is it provides the opportunity to achieve a relatively low-cost product with good aesthetics. The downside, however, is that any element of the sign that is imprinted on the first surface—such as the background color and the text—can be scathed, and sometimes the small Braille dots break off.

Before investing in any of these techniques, several details should be determined, starting with the projected volume of signage that can be produced in-house. While smaller facilities may add production to the job description of a staff member who already performs another function, larger facilities will need one full-time-equivalent staff member for every $40,000 to $60,000 in signs produced. After calculating the cost of material and labor, as well as overhead, it is reasonable to expect 25 percent to 35 percent savings with an in-house sign fabrication system over a system manufactured using an outside vendor.

Again, staff will need to police the sign system; tear down paper signs; and evaluate sign requests for appropriate terminology, size, and use. Many facilities designate an employee to handle the production of new signs but not for removing the old, outdated signs. Because this function involves refinishing walls, sign faces, and even doors, planning for removal of old signs is well worth the effort.

Lessons Learned by In-House Sign Shops

An in-house sign shop may have the tendency to be excessively accommodating and respond to every request by providing a sign. This is the same mind-set that creates overly complex policy and procedure manuals. Signs cannot solve every problem. For example, simply telling people to "keep out" may not be enough; a lock on the door may be in order.

A sign system that is easy to update can be a burden, counterintuitive as that may seem. If it takes a week to fulfill a request for a typical sign, then that time frame becomes the standard, but if Bob in the painting department takes on the job of creating the signs and his turnaround time is longer than a week, you'll find requestors' patience runs thin. Producing signs in-house also makes it hard for the responsible department to decline an ill-advised request, even if the request conflicts with established graphic standards, especially if the head of a powerful department is requesting it.

Another caution related to in-house manufacturing of signage is to resist the temptation to make a sign bigger, bolder, or red to emphasize it. Once an organization starts down this path, sign sprawl follows soon after, with each sign fighting for dominance. The result is visual pollution, with an accompanying breakdown in communication.

Like a business plan, a signage manual requires regular review and adjustment, because needs and technology change. Finally, even when in-house fabrication is available, consider using an outside vendor for major projects or items beyond the expertise of your own shop.

Codes and Standards

Health care facilities in the United States fall under the watchful eye of several building codes and standards, all of which are designed to ensure that their quality is second to none. The problem is that these regulations are constantly changing, which can make achieving compliance a bit like running alongside multiple sets of railroad tracks and trying to hop onto one moving train car after another. Each state, county, and municipality is free to adopt a different edition of the same code—or come up with its own.

Furthermore, some codes pertaining to wayfinding contradict others, and not all inspectors have current knowledge of every last iteration or understand the intent of every standard.

This chapter is not meant to serve as a definitive source on codes but rather to address some of the most common and important questions about those that relate to wayfinding.

> Design can be art. Design can be aesthetics. Design is so simple, that's why it is so complicated. Paul Rand

Before you design that first sign, then, you must contact all relevant inspection agencies, including local zoning and building agencies and fire marshals, to ascertain what version or year of which codes they enforce and to enlist their advice. What are their biggest areas of concern? What will they be looking for? What problems do they most frequently encounter? What suggestions can they make about how to proceed?

Figure 6-1 provides a list of relevant agencies and legislation, and figure 6-2 contains common questions and sources. The key to working with the various agencies is to be highly proactive: Get inspectors involved in risk assessment and design development, document the entire process, and remember that a well-designed sign system is your best defense should questions arise later.

> Good design begins with honesty, asks tough questions, comes from collaboration and from trusting your intuition.
> Freeman Thomas

Figure 6-1. Agencies or Legislation Concerning Building Codes and Standards

Agency for Healthcare Research and Quality (AHRQ) (www.ahrq.gov)
The agency is involved with several areas of data collection and standard setting. The health care field relies on AHRQ for the measurement of quality and performance, including clinical information, evidence-based practice, outcomes and effectiveness, patient safety, technology assessments, and more.

American National Standards Institute (ANSI) (www.ansi.org)
The institute is charged with setting standards on the development and manufacture of virtually every product made and process executed in the United States, from the tensile strength of bolts to the definition of Grade II Braille. According to ANSI's Web site, "As the voice of the U.S. standards and conformity assessment system, [ANSI] empowers its members and constituents to strengthen the U.S. marketplace position in the global economy while helping to assure the safety and health of consumers and the protection of the environment."[1]

Americans with Disabilities Act (ADA) (www.ada.gov)
Since the inception of the Americans with Disabilities Act, the U.S. Department of Justice (DOJ) has been the governing agency for ADA compliance. The ADA Web site addresses regulations on matters from design to enforcement issues, including signage.

Centers for Disease Control and Prevention (CDC) (www.cdc.gov)
The CDC is one of the major operating components of the U.S. Department of Health and Human Services. The CDC's involvement in wayfinding has resulted in such signage items as "Tobacco-Free Campus"; it also establishes and monitors color coding of patient care indicator signage and other standards.

The Joint Commission (www.jointcommission.org)
As the national accreditation source for Medicaid and most other federal funding, The Joint Commission establishes building and operational standards, including signage, and addresses specific issues such as ensuring that people with limited English proficiency (LEP) are provided adequate communication mechanisms.

National Fire Protection Association (NFPA) (www.nfpa.org)
As the United States' foremost authority on fire and building safety issues, NFPA sets best practices and codes that affect signage indicating area of rescue, fire evacuation, and stairwell identification (both interior and exterior), as well as signs required for elevators and many other areas.

Occupational Safety and Health Administration (OSHA) (http://osha.gov)
Under the auspices of the U.S. Department of Labor, OSHA regulates location of life safety–related signs; their appearance; and other codes, standards, and best practices. The OSHA standards include specific use of colors and a unique set of icons for messages such as biohazard warnings.

Figure 6-1. (Continued)

Underwriters Laboratories, Inc. (UL) (www.ul.com)
Underwriters Laboratories is the self-described "trusted resource across the globe for product safety certification and compliance solutions."[2] The UL guidelines regarding illuminated signage are especially critical in wayfinding projects. Even if local codes allow for illuminated signs that are not constructed in compliance with UL standards, the facility should still insist on seeing the UL label on every component.

U.S. Department of Health and Human Services (HHS) (www.hhs.gov)
Regulations from HHS will affect the posting of special notices, precautions, and other signage that is not directional in nature but is a critical element in a wayfinding system. See also state health department mandates.

U.S. Department of Transportation (DOT) (www.dot.gov)
Regulations from DOT mandate compliance with standards regarding primarily exterior signage. Several years ago, a graphic designer incorporated a custom, round stop sign into an organization's sign system lexicon that was not designed to DOT standards. In addition to the risk the organization faced of being cited by the agency for noncompliance, it also, and more importantly, risked accident or injury and perhaps subsequent legal action against any and all entities involved in the sign project, because drivers were not accustomed to the appearance of this stop sign. Be sure to also review state transportation department regulations.

Figure 6-2. Hot-Button Wayfinding Issues

Issue	Where to Look for Help
Where are mounting standards for signs defined?	ADA, state accessibility codes/standards
What defines a permanent room for accessibility standards?	ADA, state accessibility codes/standards
What constitutes a "simple typestyle" for raised and Braille signs?	ADA, state accessibility codes/standards
Where, other than elevator lobbies, must fire evacuation plans be posted?	State/local fire codes, local fire marshal
How are areas of rescue defined?	Joint Commission, state/local building codes
What size, quantity, and placement limitations apply to exterior signs?	Local building inspection department
What are the new standards associated with ADA?	ADA, state accessibility codes/standards

EXTERIOR SIGNS

For code purposes, there are two broad categories of exterior signs: on-site and off-site. Any sign that appears on property not owned by the organization is considered an off-site sign, which usually is governed by billboard regulations.

On-site Exterior Sign Codes

On-site exterior sign codes became increasingly strict starting in the 1970s in response to visual pollution created by billboards fighting for dominance. Neighborhoods all over the United States seemingly began to resemble Las Vegas in appearance until First Lady, Lady Bird Johnson became active in highway beautification. City and regional planners quickly fell in line with the effort. Sign codes originally established simply to prevent a public safety hazard in the form of driver distractions today are intent on setting and maintaining an aesthetic standard.

The general idea is to promote the use of wall-mounted signage (on a building), rather than freestanding signs, and to make the signs fewer, shorter, and smaller. Although these rules were designed with retail establishments in mind, hospitals also must adhere to restrictions. For example, one site identification sign plus a 4-square-foot directional sign saying "enter" with an arrow better serve restaurants than medical centers with their larger street frontage area, multiple curb cuts and entrances, and critical situations.

Hospitals typically seek to exempt themselves from such restrictions by applying for a zoning variance, which is costly in terms of both time (up to a year in some cases) and money. A zoning variance is a request for an exemption from the standard zoning laws. An exemption usually is predicated on the unique and urgent need of the medical facility. When seeking an exemption, to further support the application an organization is well served to present a case for financial hardship if the facility is mandated to provide compliant signage. Municipalities are reluctant to set precedents, but they will usually grant exemptions for medical facilities in service to the community.

Contact your municipality directly for information on sign and zoning codes, permits, and variance options well in advance of implementing your wayfinding program. For best results, be prepared to present your signage/wayfinding master plan in clear and easy-to-understand terms, including future phases, detailed location information, and typical sign type drawings. Extensive documentation may be required, as one organization profiled in chapter 8 discovered when applying for a variance (figure 6-3).

Department of Transportation Standards

The key document for complying with federal Department of Transportation standards is the Federal Highway Administration's *Manual on Uniform Traffic Control Devices* (*MUTCD*), which can be accessed online at www.mutcd.fhwa.dot.gov. State department of transportation agencies may mandate regulations that differ from the federal codes, but they are essentially the same and perhaps even more strict. The brief excerpts from *MUTCD* in figure 6-4 provide a sense of the regulations.

Specific guidelines cover every configuration of traffic, including yield signs and other traffic-related signage. Even on private property, the Federal Highway Administration's manual should be followed for safety's sake and to minimize legal exposure. For example, you may choose to place a stop sign on a nonstandard, decorative post, but it is strongly recommended that the sign have the appearance, shape, colors, and mounting placement dictated by *MUTCD*. Otherwise, the organization is at risk, as mentioned earlier, of a driver running the stop sign because "it did not look like one."

Figure 6-3. Sample Documentation for a Zoning Variance

Shady Grove Adventist Hospital, Rockville, Maryland, submitted this plan for exterior signage as part of its overall wayfinding program.

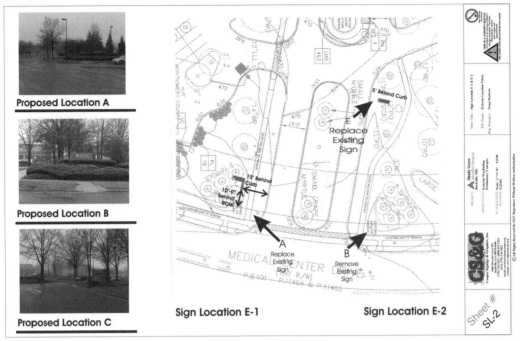

Figure 6-4. Excerpts from the Federal Highway Administration's *Manual on Uniform Traffic Control Devices*

ELIGIBILITY (SECTION 2F.01)

Standard: Specific service signs shall be defined as guide signs that provide road users with business identification and directional information for services and for eligible attractions.

- Guidance: The use of Specific Service signs should be limited to areas primarily rural in character or to areas where adequate sign spacing can be maintained.

- Option: Where an engineering study determines a need, Specific Service signs may be used on any class of highways.

- Guidance: Specific Service signs should not be installed at an interchange where the road user cannot conveniently reenter the freeway or expressway and continue in the same direction of travel.

Standard: Eligible service facilities shall comply with laws concerning the provisions of public accommodations without regard to race, religion, color, age, sex, or national origin, and laws concerning the licensing and approval of service facilities. The attraction services shall include only facilities which have the primary purpose of providing amusement, historical, cultural, or leisure activities to the public. Distances to eligible 24-hour pharmacies shall not exceed 4.8 km (3 mi) in any direction of an Interchange on the Federal-aid system.

- Guidance: Except as noted in the Option below, distances to eligible services other than pharmacies should not exceed 4.8 km (3 mi) in any direction.

Figure 6-4. (Continued)

- Option: If, within the 4.8 km (3 mi) limit, facilities for the services being considered other than pharmacies are not available or choose not to participate in the program, the limit of eligibility may be extended in 4.8 km (3 mi) increments until one or more facilities for the services being considered chooses to participate, or until 25 km (15 mi) is reached, whichever comes first.

GENERAL SERVICE SIGNS (D9 SERIES) (SECTION 2D.45)

- Support: On conventional roads, commercial services such as gas, food, and lodging generally are within sight and are available to the road user at reasonably frequent intervals along the route. Consequently, on this class of road there usually is no need for special signs calling attention to these services. Moreover, General Service signing is usually not required in urban areas except for hospitals, law enforcement assistance, tourist information centers, and camping.

- Option: General Services signs . . . may be used where such services are infrequent and are found only on an intersecting highway or crossroad.

Standard: All General Service signs and supplemental panels shall have white letters, symbols, and borders on a blue background.

- Guidance: General Service signs should be installed at a suitable distance in advance of the turn-off point or intersecting highway. States that elect to provide General Service signing should establish a statewide policy or warrant for its use, and criteria for the availability of services. Local jurisdictions electing to use such signing should follow State policy for the sake of uniformity.

- Option: Individual States may sign for whatever alternative fuels are available at appropriate locations.

[for General Service signs such as the hospital "H" trailblazer:]

Standard: General Service signs, if used at intersections, shall be accompanied by a directional message.

- Option: The General Service legends may be either symbols or word messages.

Standard: Symbols and word message General Service legends shall not be inter-mixed on the same sign. The Pharmacy (D9-20) sign shall only be used to indicate the availability of a pharmacy that is open, with a State-licensed pharmacist present and on duty, 24 hours per day, 7 days per week, and that is located within 4.8 km (3 mi) of an interchange on the Federal-aid system. The D9-20 sign shall have a 24 HR (D9-20a) plaque mounted below it.

APPLICATION OF REGULATORY SIGNS (SECTION 2B.01)

Standard: Regulatory signs shall be used to inform road users of selected traffic laws or regulations and indicate the applicability of the legal requirements. Regulatory signs shall be installed at or near where the regulations apply. The signs shall clearly indicate the requirements imposed by the regulations and shall be designed and installed to provide adequate visibility and legibility in order to obtain compliance. Regulatory signs shall be reflective or illuminated to show the same shape and similar color by both day and night, unless specifically stated otherwise in the text discussion of a particular sign or group of signs (see Section 2A.08). The requirements for sign illumination shall not be considered to be satisfied by street, highway, or strobe lighting.

CODES AND STANDARDS ON THE USE OF LANGUAGE

The federal legal authority mandating language assistance and provision of information and services in languages other than English to persons with limited English proficiency derives from Title VI of the Civil Rights Act of 1965. Any organization that receives federal financial assistance is required to comply with Title VI regulations, which are designed to help LEP persons overcome language barriers and participate meaningfully in programs, services, and benefits.

Policy guidance provided by HHS states that such an organization will be in compliance if it provides materials for eligible LEP language groups, as detailed in the Office for Civil Rights Safe Harbor Guidelines (figure 6-5).

The standards of The Joint Commission do not specifically address signage or any other aspect of wayfinding, except as it pertains to the labeling of certain areas, such as soiled/clean/sterile. However, The Joint Commission has published advice on the subject in its publications, which could be considered best practices. For example, a recent article published in *Joint Commission Perspectives* said,

> Health care facilities can be a challenge to navigate for anyone. But individuals who cannot read signage in English are at a bigger disadvantage and can become intimidated. To remedy this, many health care organizations have translated their signage into the top languages encountered by the organization.[3]

The article goes on to recommend another option to translation: the use of universal signage, which features symbols instead of words. Symbols for common hospital referents (i.e., terms that the symbols are designed to represent) can be found at the Hablamos Juntos Language Policy and Practice in Health Care Web site, www.hablamosjuntos.org/signage/symbols/default.using_symbols.asp. The symbols are ever expanding and evolving, but knowledge of the basic symbols provides a good foundation for any program.

To these recommendations, I add the following widely accepted guideline regarding wayfinding, which I call the Cooper Quotient:

> We recommend that organizations have a written visitor's guide in all languages used by 5% or more people in their service population, and give special consideration to translating wayfinding elements in emergency departments and labor/delivery/recovery units, which tend to experience the heaviest use of non-English speakers. At a facility-wide level, signs should be in all languages used by groups constituting 20% or more of the service population or should rely on an easily understood system of pictograms/icons such as those adopted by Hablamos Juntos.

Figure 6-5. Required Translations by Target LEP Group

TRANSLATION TYPE:	Number (or percent) of people in target LEP Group		
	Less than or equal to 100 persons	Less than or equal to 1,000 persons (5%) of the service population	Less than or equal to 3,000 persons (10%) of the service population
ORAL translation of written materials	✓	✓	✓
Translation of written documents		✓	✓
Translation of all documents			✓

Source: Office for Civil Rights Safe Harbor Guidelines, HHS, www.hhs.gov/ocr.

Such pictograms become increasingly important as facilities evolve to serve more than two dominant languages, because signs using four or more languages quickly become visually overwhelming and expensive (figure 6-6). This guidance should also be applied to written communications, phone translation services, and staff training. These icons supplement universal symbols such as DOT standards, OSHA-required icons, and so forth.

Of course, the language problem is not limited to non-English speakers. In a 2007 white paper called *What Did the Doctor Say? Improving Health Literacy to Protect Patient Safety*, The Joint Commission noted that effective communication is the cornerstone of patient safety.[4] Accredited organizations are explicitly encouraged to ensure understanding by patients in that segment of the American population whose literacy skills are basic (29 percent) or below (14 percent). Noting that only 33 percent of Americans have basic quantitative skills, the paper goes on to say, "when literacy collides with health care, the issue of health literacy—defined as the degree to which individuals have the capacity to obtain, process, and understand basic health information and services needed to make appropri-

ate health decisions—begins to cast a long patient safety shadow."

Among the specific recommendations the paper makes are the following:

- Ensure easy access to the health care organization by using clear wayfinding materials and signage.
- Use plain language always.

EASILY OVERLOOKED CODES AND STANDARDS

Some specific details contained in codes and standards may be overlooked. Check with your local building inspection agency for elements that may be more obscure or less obvious, such as local/state guidelines governing the accessibility of exterior signs. These codes usually dictate quantity, square footage, and placement of signs designating parking spaces, ramps, and entrances, but most codes' square footage requirements are based on the size of the actual sign face, not the entire sign or structure, and they usually refer to one side of the sign, even if the sign is double sided.

While not literally addressed by any code or standard, identification of every public door in a health care organization, indoors and outdoors, is generally considered best practice. Those doors designated for staff only should be labeled with an "Authorized Personnel Only" sign, a small investment to make to keep patients and visitors from entering an area from which they are restricted.

In addition, be aware that many municipalities have specific regulations aimed at electronic or changeable message boards.

Related to workplace safety, specific markings, colors, and pictograms are required by OSHA and should be part of your sign system. Do not rely on stickers placed on equipment by its manufacturers to achieve compliance.

Figure 6-6. Sample Signage in Multiple Languages

Listings in four or more languages can become visual pollution.

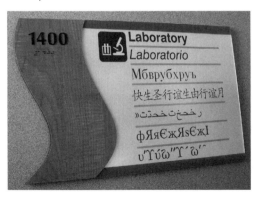

Your local fire marshal may require a number of signs related to life safety, some of them in more than one language. The goal here is to provide a helpful warning rather to threaten or frighten. For example, in a parking area, a sign that says, "NOTICE: This facility is not responsible for items left in cars" is less friendly than "Do not leave personal items unattended."

Three government agencies—HHS, CDC, and AHRQ—address wayfinding issues briefly or tangentially. Check each agency's Web site as well as with all local inspectors to determine steps for compliance.

The Department of Health and Human Services does not speak specifically to signage, leaving this topic largely to the states to regulate, but in addressing issues such as life safety, biohazard area identification, and containment, the HHS Web site does include standards for its own facilities, which may be applied to the field as well. For example:

(B.1.7) Graphics/Signage: Graphics and signage will help employees and visitors find their way through a laboratory building. Directional graphics and signage should be functional and in harmony with the architecture of the building. Signs are also important for the identification of the biohazard level of areas where biohazardous work is performed.

These standards are reinforced by the CDC on its Web site, as follows: "Standard biosafety practice requires that signage be posted on laboratory doors to alert people to the hazards that may be present within the laboratory. The biohazard sign normally includes the name of the agent, specific hazards associated with the use or handling of the agent, and contact information for the investigator."

For its part, AHRQ defines patient satisfaction measures as "reducing noise, providing more privacy, and making it easier for patients to find their way through the hospital [which] all improve patient satisfaction."[5]

AMERICANS WITH DISABILITIES ACT

The Americans with Disabilities Act sets the national standards for tactile signage, designed to provide reasonable access for both the public and employees. Accordingly, the standards apply not just to public spaces but also throughout the facility, including areas such as sterile surgical suites. See figure 6-7 for three options on tactile signage that meet federal ADA standards.

Often the act is enforced as if it were a building code, although it is not a code. However, several states have adopted as code their own version of disability standards, and interpretations vary greatly from inspector to inspector.

The DOJ has made major clarifications and modifications to ADA since its passage. On June 17, 2008, it issued a formal proposal to adopt new accessibility guidelines for the private sector and state and local governments, a long-anticipated and critical step toward updating the act.[6] The changes included in the new guidelines are in the process of being adopted, but the pace of adoption will vary from region to region.

The new guidelines, an excerpt of which appears in appendix D, include the following changes to accessible-sign specifications:

- Criteria for tactile typefaces have been updated to require a thin stroke width and widely spaced characters, without serifs or embellishments of any kind.
- Mounting height for tactile signs has changed. The baseline of tactile characters must be between 48 and 60 inches above the finished floor, slightly lower than the earlier requirement of 60 inches from the

center of the sign (figure 6-8). Some sign designs can comply with both the old and the new standard by placing the raised and Braille text at the bottom of the sign.

- A new minimum height is mandated for the appearance of visual characters. Depending on viewing distance, characters on signs mounted overhead can be as small as 2 inches if they are placed no more than 10 feet above the floor (figure 6-8). However, the minimum character size increases when signs are placed higher.

See appendix D for a more thorough explanation of these guidelines, published by the Society for Environmental Graphic Design.

More information about ADA and its regulations on signage can be found at www .access-board.gov/links/statecodes.htm and at www.segd.org.

LIFE SAFETY: NATIONAL FIRE PROTECTION ASSOCIATION

The most common wayfinding questions addressed by the NFPA concern four critical areas of fire safety signage:

- What fire evacuation/extinguisher signage is required, and where?
- What signs are required at elevators?
- What signage is required for stairwells?
- How are areas of refuge to be designated?

These areas are covered in the *NFPA 101 Life Safety Code®*. Refer to chapters 18 and 19 of the code for specific requirements for new and existing construction, respectively. The following provides a brief introduction to these areas.[7]

What fire evacuation/extinguisher signage is required, and where? No standing rule mandates that signs for floor plans or evacuation

Figure 6-7. Options for ADA-Compliant Tactile Signage

Some flexibility is given by ADA as to how tactile messages are conveyed.

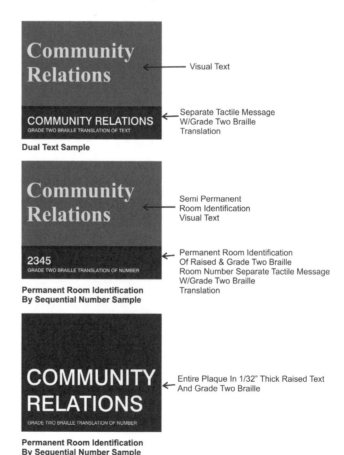

Figure 6-8. U.S. Department of Justice Guidelines on Sign Specifications

New standards for ADA mandate where a sign can be mounted. The "60 inches to the center" rule no longer applies, and the appearance of overhead lettering has more flexibility. See appendix D for more information.

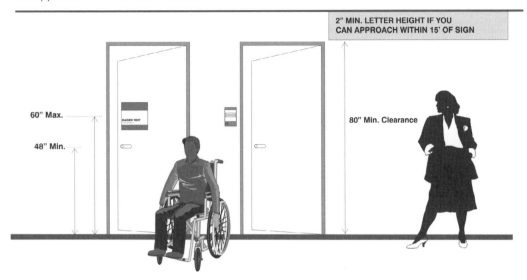

routes be provided in public areas and spaces. National Fire Prevention Association regulation 101 18.7.1.1 requires that a written plan be developed that encompasses a number of considerations. A map or figure of some sort is normally provided in that plan, with which all staff should be familiar, but these need not be posted. The code states:

> 18.7.1.1 The administration of every health care occupancy shall have, in effect and available to all supervisory personnel, written copies of a plan for the protection of all persons in the event of fire, for their evacuation to areas of refuge, and for their evacuation from the building when necessary.

Regulation 10, "Standard for Portable Fire Extinguishers," requires signs indicating the location of fire extinguishers in some circumstances, as noted:

> 6.1.3.3.2 In large rooms, and in certain locations where visual obstructions cannot be completely avoided, means shall be provided to indicate the extinguisher location.

What signs are required at elevators? Several sections of the code address the signs required at elevators. These are to be posted in the elevator lobby and must be supplemented by tactile signage. Specifically, the code states:

> 7.10.8.4 Elevators that are a part of a means of egress (see 7.2.13.1) shall have the following signs with a minimum letter height of 5/8 in. (16 mm) posted in every elevator lobby:
>
> (1) Signs that indicate that the elevator can be used for egress, including any restrictions on use
> (2) Signs that indicate the operational status of elevators
>
> A.7.10.8.4(1) These signs are to be used in place of signs that indicate that elevators are not to be used during fires. Examples of these signs include the following:
>
> In the Event of Fire, This Elevator Will Be Used by the Fire Department for Evacuation of People.
>
> PROTECTED ELEVATOR—
>
> USABLE IN EMERGENCIES

What signage is required for stairwells? The NFPA 101 criteria are very specific about the various texts, formats, and sizes that are required both inside and outside of stairwells:

> 7.2.2.5.4.1 Enclosed stairs meeting either of the following two conditions shall comply with 7.2.2.5.4.1(A) through 7.2.2.5.4.1(H):
>
> (1) The stair is a new enclosed stair serving three or more stories.
>
> (2) The stair is an existing enclosed stair serving five or more stories.
>
> 7.2.2.5.4.1(A) The stairs shall be provided with special signage within the enclosure at each floor landing.
>
> 7.2.2.5.4.1(B) The signage shall indicate the floor level.
>
> 7.2.2.5.4.1(C) The signage shall indicate the terminus of the top and bottom of the stair enclosure.
>
> 7.2.2.5.4.1(D) The signage shall indicate the identification of the stair enclosure.
>
> 7.2.2.5.4.1(E) The signage shall indicate the floor level of, and the direction to, exit discharge.
>
> 7.2.2.5.4.1(F) The signage shall be located inside the enclosure approximately 60 in. (1525 mm) above the floor landing in a position that is visible when the door is in the open or closed position.
>
> 7.2.2.5.4.1(G) The signage shall comply with 7.10.8.1 and 7.10.8.2 of this Code.
>
> 7.2.2.5.4.1(H) The floor level designation shall also be tactile in accordance with ICC/ANSI A117.1, American National Standard for Accessible and Usable Buildings and Facilities.

Stairwells do not require self-glowing signs and stripes on the floors.

How are areas of refuge to be designated? These requirements are detailed in NFPA 101 7.2.12. The criteria to identify areas of refuge are as follows:

> 7.2.12.3.5 Each area of refuge shall be identified by a sign that reads as follows:
>
> AREA OF REFUGE
>
> 7.2.12.3.5.1 The sign required by 7.2.12.3.5 shall conform to the requirements of ICC/ANSI A117.1, American National Standard for Accessible and Usable Buildings and Facilities, for such signage and shall display the international symbol of accessibility. Signs also shall be located as follows:
>
> (1) At each door providing access to the area of refuge
>
> (2) At all exits not providing an accessible means of egress, as defined in 3.3.151.1
>
> (3) Where necessary to indicate clearly the direction to an area of refuge
>
> 7.2.12.3.5.2 Signs required by 7.2.12.3.5 shall be illuminated as required for exit signs where exit sign illumination is required.
>
> 7.2.12.3.6 Tactile signage complying with ICC/ANSI A117.1, American National Standard for Accessible and Usable Buildings and Facilities, shall be located at each door to an area of refuge.

UNDERWRITERS LABORATORIES

Any lighting of signs, internal or otherwise, should include a clearly visible UL label. Underwriters Laboratories establishes a minimum standard of construction.

To have the signs and lights built to UL standards but not have a UL label present is not adequate to comply with recommendations.

SPECIALIZED SIGN CHECKLIST

In the process of developing the wayfinding master plan, make sure to account for the addition of specialized regulations, codes, and standards. For example, smaller, specialized agencies often come out with posting requirements dictating specific signs to be posted, some within a specific size, placement, and format. A department head may read an article or attend a seminar sharing the latest posting requirements and decide to proactively have new signs posted or existing signs modified in a well-meaning effort to comply. If not properly anticipated, a number of such signs will simply appear in the facility that will weaken the visual continuity of the sign system if they are not integrated appropriately.

Following is a checklist of policy and procedure signs to address in your wayfinding program:

☞ Biohazard area identification, common in clinic and especially laboratory areas

☞ Tobacco-free campus restrictions

☞ Cellular telephone policy (if the facility restricts the use of cell phones, users need to be told where to "Turn off Cell Phones" and where cell phones are permitted)

☞ After-hours admittance policy and 24-hour emergency department access (where is the "after-hours entrance"?)

☞ Emergency Medical Treatment and Active Labor Act compliance policies

☞ Physician assistants (when and where are they administering care?)

☞ Separate billing policies (such as x-rays that will be billed through a third party, not the hospital)

☞ Health Insurance Portability and Accountability Act and patient confidentiality reminders to staff and visitors

☞ "Medicare/Medicaid accepted" (and other statements on insurance that need to be posted)

☞ "No concealed weapons" (some state laws require this message to be posted)

☞ Triage policy (e.g., "Patients will be seen in the order of medical need, not order of arrival")

☞ Hand hygiene (a recent, yet important, guide; what is your current policy?)

☞ Children's visiting policy, usually unique to each facility (conveyed in a friendly, positive manner)

☞ "If you are under the weather . . ." (then what?)

☞ "Notify the technologist if you think you may be pregnant" (post this message prominently in imaging areas)

Department head surveys administered early in the wayfinding planning process will generate a very good list of the signs required for each area. It is important, however, to devise a system to accommodate new policies and procedures as they are needed.

As stated earlier, codes and standards are fluid, open for interpretation and updates. Make compliance a core design parameter, but even better, be proactive to address the intention of the code, not just minimal compliance levels.

Most of the precepts reviewed to this point of the book apply to a wide range of medical facilities but are specific to acute care settings. Chapter 7 considers some unique aspects of non-acute care facilities, specifically ambulatory care clinics, medical office buildings, extended care facilities, retail space, and parking structures.

REFERENCES

1. American National Standards Institute, "About ANSI Overview" (accessed November 22, 2009), http://www.ansi.org/about_ansi/overview/overview.aspx?menuid=1.

2. Underwriters Laboratories, Inc., "Welcome to Underwriters Laboratories" (accessed November 22, 2009), http://www.ul.com/global/eng/pages/.

3. The Joint Commission, "Promoting Effective Communication—Language Access Services in Health Care," *Joint Commission Perspectives,* 28 (2): 8–11.

4. The Joint Commission, *What Did the Doctor Say? Improving Health Literacy to Protect Patient Safety* (accessed November 23, 2009), http://www.jointcommission.org/NR/rdonlyres/D5248B2E-E7E6-4121-8874-99C7B4888301/0/improving_health_literacy.pdf.

5. Agency for Healthcare Research and Quality, "Transforming Hospitals, Designing for Safety and Quality" (accessed November 23, 2009), http://www.ahrq.gov/qual/transform.pdf.

6. U.S. Access Board, *ADA Accessibility Guidelines for Buildings and Facilities (ADAAG)* (accessed November 23, 2009), http://www.access-board.gov/adaag/html/adaag.htm.

7. Personal correspondence with Robert Solomon, PE, engineer, National Fire Prevention Association. This information does not constitute a formal interpretation pursuant to NFPA regulations or professional consultation or services.

CHAPTER 7

Specialized Facilities

ost of this book deals with wayfinding in hospitals for an obvious reason: Hospitals pose the most complex logistical challenge in health care. And most of the information presented thus far applies, with some common-sense modifications, to the full range of hospitals: large, small, urban, rural, teaching, specialized, and community hospitals and tertiary care centers. It also applies, for the most part, to other health care facilities.

However, ambulatory care clinics, medical office buildings (MOBs), extended care facilities, retail space (e.g., medical malls), and parking structures do present the wayfinding committee or task force with some special considerations, as does the medical campus as a whole.

> Design is directed toward human beings. To design is to solve human problems by identifying them and executing the best solution. Ivan Chermayeff

THE UNIFIED MEDICAL CAMPUS

Earlier chapters have demonstrated that signage serves more than one purpose: In addition to helping people find their way around, it also helps the health care provider project a certain image. This is true whether or not you intend to do so, so you are better off taking image into account when you design your wayfinding program.

Whether you are a small and rural facility striving to position yourself as a provider of more personal, compassionate care than might be available in the big city; an urban facility boasting sophisticated technology and board-certified medical staff; or a

> Design is a plan for arranging elements in such a way as best to accomplish a particular purpose. Charles Eames

suburban facility promoting a specialty service, your lexicon of signs should reflect your mission and goals.

Of course, many people will go to the closest facility in an emergency or to the facility recommended by their physician for elective procedures. But as organizations resort more and more to marketing and direct community outreach to set themselves apart from the competition, consumers are playing a more active role in the selection process.

Health plans, employers, governments, and health care providers themselves are working hard to provide reliable, objective information about quality and, increasingly, costs on the Internet and in other media. But these efforts are still in their infancy, leaving many consumers to rely primarily on general reputation, fleeting impressions, and second- or third-hand experiences—in short, image.

Physicians, whether considered customers, competitors, or partners of the enterprise—most likely, all three—are less influenced by image (although still plenty susceptible to their surroundings). But if they have a choice among health care providers at which to admit or treat patients, the ease with which they can get in and out of the provider's facilities can become a major factor in their decision making. Hence, signage is a key component to that facilitation.

What else do signs provide? Executed well, they lend cohesiveness to a medical campus. As a health care organization grows physically—often lurching into the future, rather than progressing in an orderly fashion—the sense of a unified campus with unified architecture and signage can easily get lost. Without a master wayfinding plan, the different buildings, each with its special function, funds, and champions, can end up fighting each other for visual dominance. Signs can help make the whole more than the sum of its individual parts.

Consider the following questions in determining the effectiveness of your medical campus signage:

- How is your campus delineated from the rest of the streetscape? Is it clear that it *is* a campus? Is it clear how to access it from every direction?
- How does traffic flow in and around the campus? Does this flow make the best use of the site? Perhaps you want to have visitors drive by the wellness center even if

that is not the shortest route to their destination.
- Is each building and/or entrance associated with a specific parking area—and is this association clear to visitors? Or does a lot of stressful milling about take place as people search for the spot closest to the first building they see, only to find out it is not the right access point for their destination? Are areas reserved for physicians, staff, and emergencies clearly marked?
- Are people told to look for the "cancer center" when the signs say "Smith Oncology Pavilion"? Remember the importance of straightforward and consistent terminology.

AMBULATORY CARE CLINICS

To patients, clinics and urgent care centers are all about convenience and cost. These facilities are often frequented by the uninsured, the underinsured, and those without a regular primary care practitioner because they are easier and cheaper to access than the hospital emergency department. If your organization has affiliated clinics and urgent care centers, you should extend your signage and branding to the premises as far as is practical. This extension of identification is easier to accomplish on hospital or health system property, where the parent organization can exert tighter control; if the property is leased, make sure that the lease agreement is friendly to the wayfinding program.

Whether affiliated or independent, ambulatory care facilities—including surgicenters—face many of the same wayfinding problems as do acute care facilities, only with smaller budgets and tighter spaces. Fortunately, codes and standards generally are less stringent for these facilities, as long as they are compliant with basic elements such as the Americans with Disabilities Act and fire and building codes.

MEDICAL OFFICE BUILDINGS

Whether referred to as medical office buildings, professional offices, or medical pavilions, MOBs have a way of popping up on a hospital campus without clear identification. Patients looking for their doctor's office may have several similar structures to choose from, with little or no guidance to help differentiate them.

One way to make it easier for visitors to find a particular building—and easier for you to direct them—is to assign and use a regular street address (figure 7-1) in addition to whatever formal name the building may carry. In addition, make sure the address is as prominent as the name on the signage. Another way to facilitate wayfinding here is to clearly label a specific parking lot or area as belonging to the building and direct people to it. This approach is more difficult, but not impossible, when one or more MOBs are physically attached to the main hospital.

Again, if the building is owned by a third party and you did not negotiate wayfinding issues before signing the lease, you will have limited control over signage and building directories. Directories can be a particularly thorny issue. For aesthetic and growth purposes, conventional wisdom says to leave 20 percent of the overall space blank, but this guideline does not tell you how big the directory will actually need to be. Southeast Gynecology may need to list five doctors, while Harold Smith, MD, in suite 210 may need only a single strip.

Your best approach is to allocate three strips of text for each projected tenant—one for the firm or group name and two for physicians' names—and try to enforce the limitation. If extra space is available, you can use it to showcase the building logo, display a floor plan (as shown in figure 7-2), or indicate where restrooms are located.

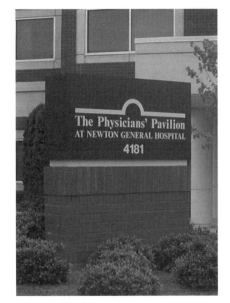

Figure 7-1. Sample Signage with Street Address

In today's world of navigational systems and online tools, having an address on exterior signs is a good idea in support of those systems.

Figure 7-2. Sample Building Directory

Use extra space to display a floor plan.

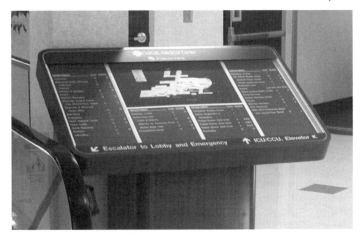

Signage at suite entrances themselves must be easy to update. Even the most stable practice can find itself with new partners or information to impart, and physicians will not readily understand costs and delays associated with updating. Design a sign program that highlights the suite number and limits the tenant to a single sign or insert of a consistent, reasonable size. Let the practice know that less is more when it comes to effective signage but that it can list whatever it wants—as long as it fits in the space allocated, say 11" × 11".

Figure 7-3 shows a simple 8½" × 11" card stock insert that can be reproduced on any inkjet printer and updated for pennies in a few minutes. Elements that are frequently posted on suite signs include:

- Suite number
- Practice name
- Physicians' names
- Specialties
- Hours
- Physician assistants' names
- Logo
- Delivery policies
- Separately marked entrances for well/sick patients
- Credit cards/insurance accepted

Inside the suites, the particular specialty will dictate the space and wayfinding needs: A pediatrician will want a play space, for example, and an optometrist will need room for a retail display.

Regardless of the specialty, however, lobbies are almost always characterized by sensory overload—aging magazines, check-in information, a television, and a constant flow of traffic. The more upfront planning you can do to accommodate these needs, the better will be the wayfinding outcome, especially in terms of patient satisfaction, as first impressions are often indelible. Note that

the TV screen can be used to communicate all kinds of care information, policies, and promotional material along with whatever televised program is airing.

A physician's office is all about efficiency: patients in, through, and out. The overall effect should be professional without being impersonal or cold, and this recommendation extends to the signage. For example, "Help us keep your cost down by being on time for every appointment; a fee may be charged for missed appointments" gets the message across without being threatening.

Once patients pass through the door that separates the lobby from the examination and treatment areas, they usually are escorted, so minimal directional signage is needed until the visit is over. At that point, most offices expect patients to find their own way back out, so exits (and paths back to the reception desk to make follow-up appointments and to pay) had better be clearly marked.

Office staff may wish to supplement signage with their own visual cues. At the exam room doors, for example, chart boxes and color-coded plastic flags or paddles display the room status: occupied, ready for the physician, and so forth (figure 7-4). Each office devises its own system.

Steer clear, however, of offering too many messages inside exam rooms. Time spent waiting for the physician is often filled with anxiety or spent focusing on the problem

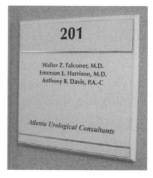

Figure 7-3. Sample Suite Signage with Card Stock Insert
Suite signs need to be easy and economical to update.

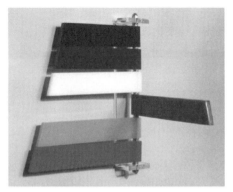

Figure 7-4. Signage as Interior Accent: Color-Coded Plastic Flags
Clean, concise signage can be an interior accent while also being functional.

that brought the patient there; these are not "teachable moments." Any critical information posted on exam room walls and counters should be repeated elsewhere.

EXTENDED CARE FACILITIES

Extended care facilities, whether freestanding or attached to a hospital, are a true hybrid: They are caregiving environments that are also residences. Whether intended or not, signage contributes to the impression of a nurturing, home-like environment or a warehouse for the elderly, especially when families are shopping for a residence for a loved one.

In contrast to that of acute care facilities, the visitor volume at extended care facilities is minimal and behavior often repetitive, so directional information is subdued: concise, understated, and helpful without being insistent. Instead of directing hurried strangers, its primary role is to gently remind residents who may have dementia and other disorienting conditions.

When designing patient room signage, keep in mind that the room is someone's home address and should be treated with commensurate dignity.

RETAIL SPACE

Medical malls are a recent innovation that seems to have staying power. Along with health care services such as physical therapy, blood centers, outpatient laboratories, clinics, and service line outposts, medical malls provide a range of convenience services, including:

- Gift shops
- Pharmacies
- Optical shops
- Durable medical equipment shops
- Fitness/wellness centers
- Branch banks
- Coffee shops (even food courts)
- Day care (for well and under-the-weather children)
- Adult day care

Such services are primarily offered for employees and patients but also look to extend their reach as far as possible to the general public. Accordingly, wayfinding and promotion are both important elements of their signage programs, as in a strictly retail facility (figure 7-5).

Figure 7-5. Sample Signage for a Retail Space
Retail areas require more than simple identification: They need to be image driven and to self-promote the business.

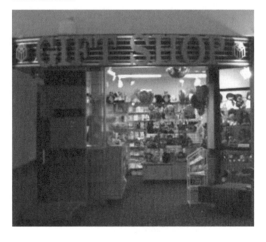

The trick is to strike an aesthetic and a practical balance between the retail and the medical aspects of the mall. The parent organization has limited control of the retail sign lexicon—it is hard to tell McDonald's that it cannot display its logo. Indeed, large logos, back-lighted menu boards, and expansive curtain walls are the norm in retail, so it is best to contain these establishments in a specific area when possible.

Another recent development is almost the reverse phenomenon: Instead of locating retail businesses in medical malls, medical facilities and related services—chiropractic or physical therapy, for example—are locating in strictly retail environments like the traditional shopping center. Express clinics are becoming more common in malls, sometimes situated in pharmacies.

To be successful in this kind of setting, you may need to bulk up your current signage or branding with retail-like images and easy-to-spot logos to make a strong visual impact. You are at the mercy of the mall's own standards here, so make sure they are compatible with your mission and purpose before signing a lease, and avoid abstract medical terms consumers will not instantly recognize. For example, a term like *orthopedic center* may be less public-friendly than *sports medicine center*.

PARKING STRUCTURES

Today it seems there is never enough parking available. Whether called lots, decks, ramps, or garages, parking areas are expensive and difficult to maintain. If enclosed, they are typically dark and uninviting and smell of gas fumes. People do not feel safe in them, and often they are not.

Wayfinding cannot resolve all these concerns, but making it easy for people to find and navigate parking structures can enhance the success of your health care facility. Introducing colors, environmental graphics, and additional lighting can help make the parking experience feel less fraught with anxiety. Curved panels with reflective copy (figure 7-6) also help drivers to read critical information when making quick decisions.

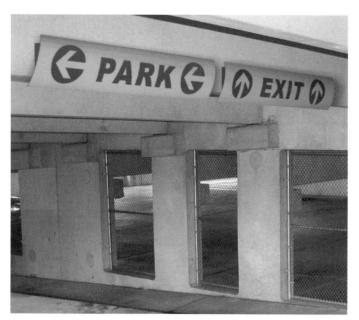

Figure 7-6. Sample Signage for User-Friendly Parking
Mounting curved panels with reflective copy helps provide better line of sight and headlight illumination, even in poorly lighted decks.

Safety features like scream alarms and monitors can help make parking a more secure environment. But how do you let people know about those features without scaring them? A sign reading "NOTICE: This area is being monitored for your safety" is a positive message you might consider using.

People parking at your facilities for the first time will have a lot of questions. It is the job of your wayfinding committee to make sure they get answers to all of them, quickly and clearly:

- Is there valet parking? What does it cost? Where do I pay?
- If the lot is remote, do you provide shuttle service to the main building(s)? Where do I board the shuttle?
- Is there an overflow lot? If so, where is it, and how do I get there?
- How can I remember where I parked? (You can place printed cards in containers attached to the columns with the level, aisle, row number, etc., as shown in figure 7-7. But you will need to keep stock on hand.)

- What path do I follow to get to the elevator, stairway, or building entrance?
- Where is the hospital entrance?
- Who is responsible if an item is stolen from my car?
- Is there a time limit? A closing time?
- Can I get my parking ticket validated? If so, where?
- If the system features prepay, where is the pay station?
- I'm leaving now. How do I get back to Main Street?

When designing signage for parking facilities, steer clear of visual obstacles. One of the biggest challenges is figuring out how to overcome poor lines of sight and low ceilings in the form of concrete T-bars, or precast concrete supports that form the exposed underside of the floor above. One suggestion is to install warning lights at blind intersections and clearance beams (sometimes called "headache bars," such as that shown in figure 7-8). These beams should be free to swing and made durable enough to absorb daily antenna whipping.

Figure 7-7. Sample Information Station within a Parking Structure
This station is equipped with containers at key locations providing a printed card that the visitor can take to help her remember where she parked.

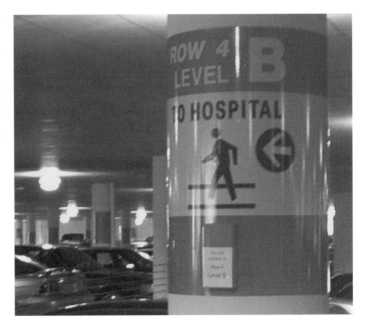

Figure 7-8. Sample Clearance Beam within a Parking Structure
Signage can help address legal issues such as clearances and other cautions.

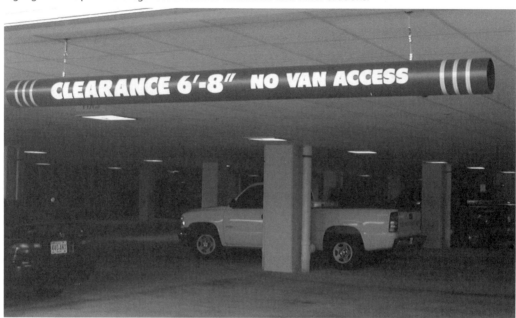

Whether you are planning a wayfinding program for a 1,200-bed acute care hospital or a physician's office, the principle of simple, clear communications is the same: Provide an environment that is inviting and easy for your clients—the patients—to use. The rewards are improved customer satisfaction, increased efficiency, and a more positive workplace—one dedicated to healing.

Chapter 8 presents real-world scenarios from the wayfinding client's perspective and addresses needs that are common to many facilities nationwide. The emphasis is on stating the problem and exploring how each client addressed it.

Case Examples

The health care wayfinding case examples in this chapter are designed to illustrate real-world applications of the information in this book. They are merely representative of the range of projects and goals that can be accomplished.

The examples are drawn from Grady Memorial Hospital, Atlanta; University Health Systems of Eastern Carolina and East Carolina University, Greenville, North Carolina; St. Anthony's Medical Center, St. Louis, Missouri; Shady Grove Adventist Hospital, Rockville, Maryland; Tift Regional Medical Center, Tifton, Georgia; Princeton Community Hospital, Princeton, West Virginia; Rockdale Medical Center, Conyers, Georgia; The Finley Hospital, Dubuque, Iowa; and the American Cancer Society's Hope Lodge locations in Georgia, North Carolina, and South Carolina.

The examples are arranged roughly in order of size of organization, from largest to smallest. The data provided are as of 2009. Our heartfelt thanks to each organization for allowing us to share its story.

COHESION IN ANY LANGUAGE: GRADY MEMORIAL HOSPITAL, GRADY HEALTH SYSTEM, ATLANTA*

As the flagship of the largest public, not-for-profit health system in the southeastern United States, Grady Memorial Hospital—built in 1958 and expanded every decade thereafter—is massive, with 953 beds, 2 million square feet, 22 stories, 11 wings, 7 public elevator banks, and 6 public entrances.

At a Glance
Established: 1958
Beds: 953
Population served: 2.8 million
Inpatient admissions: 25,763
Outpatient visits: 771,322
Employees: 5,088
Square footage: 2 million

Like Atlanta itself, Grady's patient population is widely diverse: As identified by the system's Department of Multicultural Affairs, major languages spoken by Grady's limited English proficiency population include Spanish, Mandarin, French, Bengali, Vietnamese, Amharic, Russian, Somali, and Arabic.

Under the direction of its wayfinding consultant, Grady began a project in fall 2006 to create a comprehensive new signage and wayfinding plan. The plan was conceived to bring cohesion to the hospital structure and, ultimately, to the system's ancillary buildings.

---

*Our thanks to George Smith, architectural project manager, Grady Health System Facilities Development, for providing this information.

As the plan took shape, some key decisions were made:

- The building would be subdivided into towers, named after the compass points; wing designations would keep their existing names.
- New signs would be color coded and include the Hablamos Juntos symbols. (The health system had helped to develop these symbols as a participant in the Hablamos Juntos/Society for Environmental Graphic Design (SEGD)/Robert Wood Johnson Foundation study to develop universal symbols for health care.)
- Elevator banks would be named by tower location, replacing a non-intuitive alphanumeric naming convention.
- The proposed system would be easy to maintain.

Starting in August 2007, Grady's emergency department (ED) served as a beta site, testing prototypes of the signs. A plan to move forward with permanent signage hospital-wide is currently in development.

In addition to meeting or exceeding Culturally and Linguistically Appropriate Services standards and Americans with Disabilities Act; Title VI; and other federal, local, and accreditation mandates, the new signage system reflects Grady's ongoing efforts—including continuing collaboration with Hablamos Juntos and SEGD—to eliminate barriers to health care access and to encourage culturally and linguistically appropriate services for the diverse population.

Grady deals with multilingual needs by using icons and pictograms in static signs and employing multilingual electronic units in heavy traffic areas.

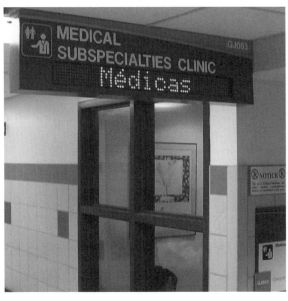

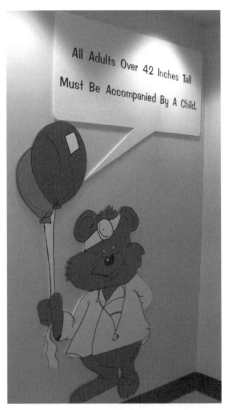

In the heavily trafficked ED, Grady set aside a play area for younger children and had some fun with the graphics.

A comprehensive room-numbering system was established for

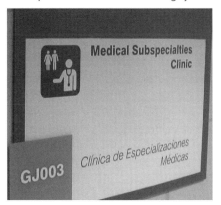

raised lettering and Grade II Braille compliance while allowing for an easy-to-update card stock insert system in two languages.

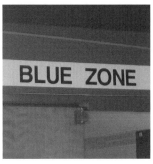

Color-coded zones help orient visitors in a very complex environment. Each sign has a color accent to reinforce the scheme.

Defining areas by color, compiling a comprehensive alphanumeric classification system, and assigning room numbers was a key to the success of wayfinding for Grady.

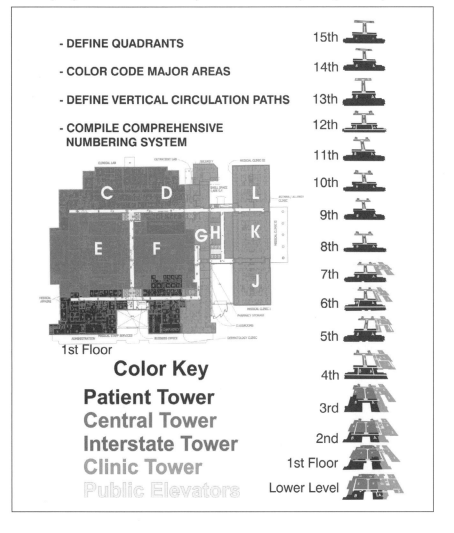

COOPERATION YIELDS RESULTS: UNIVERSITY HEALTH SYSTEMS OF EASTERN CAROLINA AND EAST CAROLINA UNIVERSITY, GREENVILLE, NORTH CAROLINA*

At a Glance
Established: 1951
Beds: 861
Population served: 1.3 million
Inpatient admissions: 34,588
Outpatient visits: 276,405
Employees: 5,588
Square footage: Combined campus of seven square miles, known locally as the Medical District

Two highly regarded health care providers. One campus. In a nutshell, that is the problem that brought University Health Systems of Eastern Carolina (UHS) and East Carolina University (ECU) to its wayfinding consultant in 2008 for a solution.

For more than 30 years, UHS's flagship hospital, Pitt County Memorial Hospital (PCMH), has shared a 100-acre parcel in Greenville, North Carolina, with ECU's Health Sciences Division. With 861 beds, PCMH, the teaching hospital for ECU's Brody School of Medicine, is the state's fifth largest hospital and home to the East Carolina Heart Institute of Pitt County Memorial Hospital. The ECU Health Sciences Division includes the Brody School of Medicine, the East Carolina Heart Institute at East Carolina University, the colleges of nursing and allied health sciences, and a new school of dentistry.

Throughout their 30-plus-year partnership, ECU and UHS have planned wayfinding independently, a system that has produced signage that advances each organization's distinct brand but gives the campus an inconsistent look.

To better serve patients and their families, as well as physicians and medical students working in the Medical District, UHS and ECU agreed last year to jointly develop a master plan for campus wayfinding.

Integrating campus signage posed several challenges: to preserve and strengthen each entity's brand, maintain cost-efficiency, and develop a scalable plan that could be tailored to the needs of individual buildings.

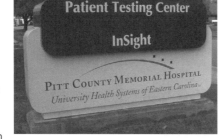

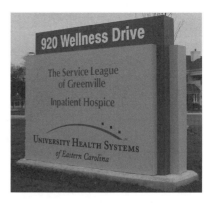

Old signage (on the left) was replaced with new signage (on the right) that incorporates a street address and updated colors. The old mounting base was used, saving substantial cost.

*Our thanks to Anissa Davenport, vice president, Strategic Development, University Health Systems of Eastern Carolina, for providing this information.

Other issues needed resolving, too: the lack of distinguishing signage on the Medical District's perimeter, outdated signage designs that featured building names more prominently than addresses, and the need to integrate with the city of Greenville's own wayfinding initiatives. Further muddling the signage is the fact that, though the ECU Health Sciences Campus and PCMH each consist of several buildings, each organization uses a single, central address.

The wayfinding consultant rose to the challenge by helping UHS and ECU develop a design that lays the foundation for a phased, multiyear effort to integrate wayfinding across the medical campus. Details of the plan include the following:

- A standard sign design that, through its use of color, reinforces ECU's and UHS's respective brands. Teal will be the dominant color on UHS building signs, while ECU signs will feature purple.
- A higher profile for street addresses, which will occupy the top line on exterior building signage.
- Large brick cornerstones marking strategic entrances to the Medical District.

- Incorporation of the city's existing signage priorities.
- Guidelines for scaling plans up or down, making it easier to export plans to other UHS and ECU facilities.
- Preservation of each organization's current practices for the most local signs.

While full implementation of the plan will take several years, new and replacement signs are already reflecting its principles. In October 2008, UHS opened a new inpatient hospice facility. Signage there follows the consultant's design, as do placards at the new East Carolina Heart Institute at Pitt County Memorial Hospital.

Straightforward vista signage delineates the hospital entrance from hundreds of other entrances.

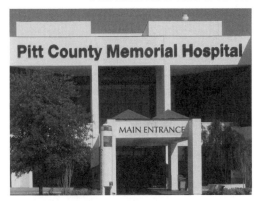

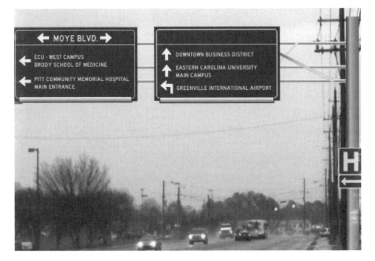

In development with the state and city departments of transportation (DOT) is over-the-highway signage for the hospital, the university, and key destinations in the city.

Large cornerstone elements clearly define and welcome visitors to the seven-square-mile Medical District. The elements incorporate water features, flags, extensive masonry, and signs to delineate the various components of the district.

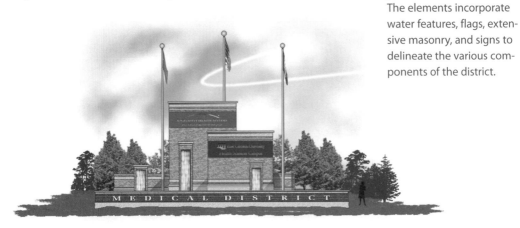

At key portals to the site, freestanding welcome center elements convey information on behalf of the Medical District and the local chamber of commerce.

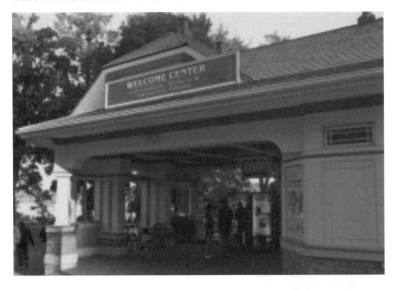

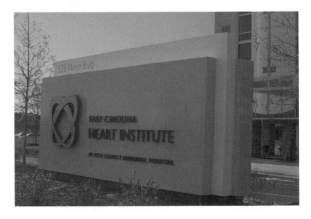

In collaboration with the architect, the wayfinding consultant implemented this site identification sign as a beta test site for the entire exterior sign program.

PATRON SAINT LEADS THE WAY: ST. ANTHONY'S MEDICAL CENTER, ST. LOUIS, MISSOURI*

After more than 100 years of service to the St. Louis metropolitan area, St. Anthony's Medical Center was remaking itself: Changes in all facets of performance included a complete overhaul of signage and wayfinding dictated by patient complaints, lost visitor reports, and visual inspection. The goals were to create a visual hierarchy that brings signage in line with more contemporary standards; develop attractive, utilitarian signage that projects the organization's image; and improve patient satisfaction scores.

Plans were drawn up to start with the interior of the main hospital building, followed by implementation in off-site buildings and, ultimately, external signage both on and off the main campus. A newly remodeled first floor would serve as a pilot test site. The wayfinding consultant decided to incorporate an award-winning signage system that had been used successfully in other organizations around the United States, incorporating St. Anthony's image on the major and most important directional signs.

Adapting lessons learned from the pilot, the next phases incorporated the following features:

- Color-coordinated signage matching distinctive colors assigned to each floor
- Large, wall-mounted floor numbers that included secondary directories in plain view of all elevators
- A series of ceiling- and wall-mounted signs routing visitors from the parking lot to the correct entrances and elevators for the connected medical office building (MOB) and to the main hospital lobby, and routing them from one facility to the next

At a Glance

Established: 1900

Beds: 767

Population served: 714,935

Inpatient admissions: 30,829

Outpatient visits: 408,145

Employees: more than 4,000

Square footage: 1,099,107

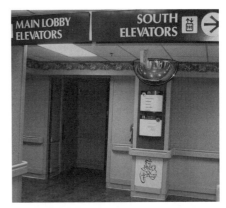

A complete interior signage system was color coded per floor to aid visitors in finding their way.

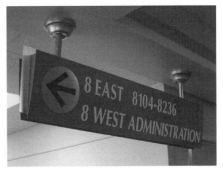

Old terminology of *East* and *West* was refined and retained in the new wayfinding program.

---

*Our thanks to Carl Martinson, senior vice president, Marketing (retired), St. Anthony's Medical Center, for providing this information.

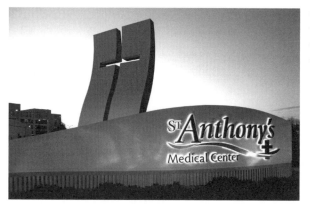

Over the course of about three years, the medical center completely renovated all interior signage and way-finding in all its facilities and partially installed a newly designed exterior wayfinding concept. The program evolved into an entire streetscape redevelopment project, including landscaping, grading, new signage, and large sculptural crosses. All of the organization's objectives were met, including an increase in patient satisfaction scores with regard to patients' feeling of comfort, ease of getting around, and overall impression of the facility.

- Large, building-mounted and freestanding off-site signs to direct attention to St. Anthony's three urgent care centers and to indicate where in those buildings physician's offices were located
- A large, building-mounted sign highlighting the new women's health services component of a facility that also housed an outpatient surgery center, a senior center, and physician's offices, which were announced on a freestanding yard sign near the entrance to the parking area
- Topography modification, landscaping, and new identity sculptures and entrance portals to soften and define the entire campus, which had grown haphazardly over the years.

In a collaborative project with a local children's hospital, St. Anthony's provides a dedicated children's ED.

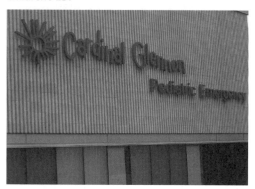

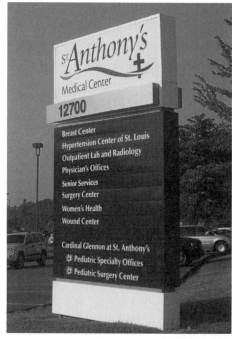

Freestanding signage with multi-tenant spaces allows street exposure for key elements in the medical plaza.

PATIENT-DRIVEN ENVIRONMENTS: SHADY GROVE ADVENTIST HOSPITAL, ROCKVILLE, MARYLAND*

Shady Grove Adventist Hospital, located in the Washington, D.C., suburb of Rockville, Maryland, embarked on a $99 million expansion project that would not only increase the facility's capacity and services but also redefine the campus and the way hospital services were accessed by patients and visitors. Prior to the addition of its new tower, a single visitor entry point to the campus provided access to all patient services. The addition of the new tower essentially created a new entrance for patients and visitors accessing the services in that tower. The combination of the new tower and the issue of a single access point led to the establishment of a new exterior wayfinding system.

In addition to addressing the exterior issues, the hospital made a commitment to the Planetree philosophy of patient-centered care and a healing environment for the new tower, creating the need for a new signage system that would complement the interior architectural elements put into place. A firm was hired at this point to serve as the wayfinding and signage design consultants for both the exterior and interior phases of the project.

Working with the Adventist staff, the firm designed a comprehensive signage system with eight different design schemes to provide the facility's management team with options to meet their perceived needs. Once a final design was approved, extensive documentation was produced and prepared for variances that would be required by the local Rockville authorities for permitting and implementing

At a Glance
Established: 1979
Beds: 275
Population served: more than 3 million
Inpatient admissions: 21,170
Outpatient visits: 158,018
Employees: 1,900
Square footage: 865,000

the new signage system. Upon presentation of the documentation, the local officials granted the variances, and the new exterior wayfinding system and temporary signs for construction were put into place.

While the exterior signage package was in production, the wayfinding design firm worked with the Adventist team to develop an interior system that would complement the Planetree interior design philosophy and serve as the second phase of the project. Construction documents were produced, and production of the interior signage was contracted to another vendor, which ultimately defaulted on the contract. The original firm was brought back in to complete fabrication and installation of the signage.

Upon completion of the new tower, the addition of a new parking structure—the third phase of the project—was begun. With the addition of the new parking structure, additional exterior signage was required, and changes to the newly implemented exterior system were made to improve the visitors' experience by providing the best route to their destination.

The final phase of the project consisted of retrofitting the interior signage system of the

---

*Our thanks to Kris Hakanson, director, Service Excellence, Shady Grove Adventist Hospital, for providing this information.

existing buildings to accommodate all of the moves and changes that had occurred over the previous four years due to the addition of the new tower and renovations to the previously existing areas. The signage system for this portion of the building will be compatible with the system implemented in the new tower as well as with the Planetree concepts. This final phase is vital to help guide visitors to their destination and to tie the entire campus together.

Changeable inserts, accented with a metallic counter surface, were used in phase 1 of the interior program.

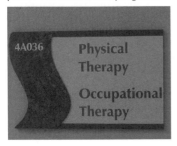

One arrow per panel makes clearer which listings are to be found in which direction.

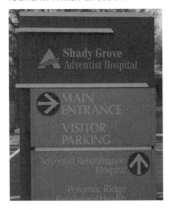

Shady Grove Children's Hospital is a "hospital inside of a hospital" that has its own identity while working within the corporate branding.

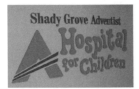

After several alternate exterior concepts were reviewed, a multipanel, multicolor program evolved.

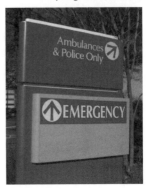

The initial rollout features changeable inserts on a variety of directional modules.

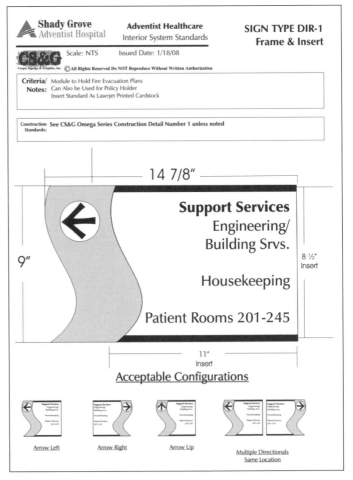

BUILDING ON STRENGTHS TO OVERCOME DEFICIENCIES: TIFT REGIONAL MEDICAL CENTER, TIFTON, GEORGIA*

In 2000, two separate but related events took place at Tift Regional Medical Center, a 191-bed regional, not-for-profit hospital serving twelve counties in south central Georgia. First, a new medical tower was added, including several new elevators, which affected a majority of medical services provided on the main campus. Second, a new imaging campaign, complete with new logo, was initiated.

The combined impact of these two developments made clear the need for Tift to analyze its existing signage and wayfinding systems. Tift leadership did not take long to realize that a new system was needed—and that redoing the entire facility was financially out of the question. Instead, a wayfinding consultant introduced a new, modified version of the current system that would build on it strengths, bring it in line with Americans with Disabilities Act (ADA) requirements, and allow for easy updating.

Here is how Tift accomplished it.

Problem: Exterior signage was out of date and not uniform. The hospital had made a significant investment in some new interior signage but was not getting support from the vendor.
Solution: The new wayfinding program featured a comprehensive sign system that unified the facility, inside and out; it built on and added to existing interior signage, and it replaced exterior signs.

Problem: The new construction would dramatically shift the way the facility was used.

At a Glance
Established: 1941
Beds: 191
Population served: 250,400
Inpatient admissions: 9,770
Outpatient visits: 121,045
Employees: 1,193
Square footage: 675,568

As the facility evolved, the elevators and wings would have no comprehensive nomenclature.
Solution: A new methodology was developed using a quadrant system tied to vertical circulation paths. Under this methodology, horizontal areas, or "quadrants," were established to tell people what wing or area they need to find and which of the corresponding elevators, unique to those areas, they need to take. For example, the "east wing" relates to the "east wing elevator." This methodology was reinforced with traditional directional signage with an expanded system of icons.

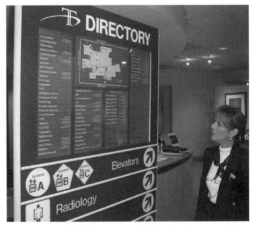

The main lobby directory can be read on several levels, by major area listings, by secondary listings, or by floor plan.

*Our thanks to Chris Efaw, director, Marketing, Tift Regional Medical Center, for providing this information.

Problem: There were now multiple elevators with no specific plan for their use and designation.

Solution: Preferred paths to various destinations were determined, with an emphasis on providing directions via specific elevators. The usage of these paths was reinforced in staff training, signage, map handouts, and posted maps.

Problem: The new corporate logo needed to be properly showcased both on-site and regionally.

Solution: The new exterior signage served as an effective platform to display the new branding, becoming an integral part of the marketing effort.

Problem: The cost of implementation was a major concern.

Solution: By updating rather than replacing the interior signage, Tift reduced costs and made a smooth transition to the new program.

Problem: Not all signs were ADA compliant.

Solution: New signage was designed to be compliant with ADA and numerous other codes and standards.

Problem: Satellite facilities were not visually linked to the main campus.

Solution: All signs, on- and off-site, were designed to have a similar look that would accommodate both heavy-hitting, retail-oriented facilities and lower-key core facilities.

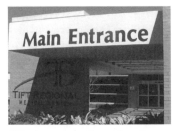

What was once the only entrance to the hospital became officially designated as the "Main Entrance," with updated signage.

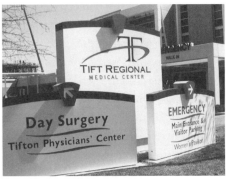

Key cornerstones became more sculptural to break up information that needed to be quickly communicated.

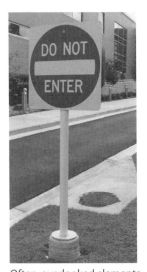

Often-overlooked elements—like DOT signage with a decorative concrete base (to reduce lawn care damage to the post)—provide a unified appearance.

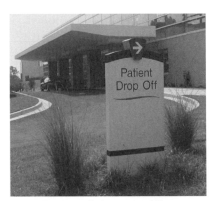

Even small elements of the streetscape were integrated into the wayfinding lexicon.

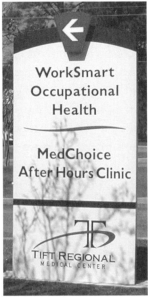

Off-site facilities are visually unified by appearance using Tift-associated colors and the Tift logo.

QUALITY CARE CLOSE TO HOME: PRINCETON COMMUNITY HOSPITAL, PRINCETON, WEST VIRGINIA*

Princeton Community Hospital identified and addressed the following wayfinding problems:

The existing signage was not uniform and was dramatically out of date. The new wayfinding system used a comprehensive exterior and interior sign system to provide a unified appearance throughout the facility. The interior was two tiered to achieve a higher aesthetic level in public spaces and a more basic variation in administrative spaces. Americans with Disabilities Act–compliant signage was implemented facility-wide.

> At a Glance
> Established: 1970
> Beds: 188
> Population served: 250,000
> Inpatient admissions: 8,075
> Outpatient visits: 172,568
> Employees: 817
> Square footage: more than 400,000

New construction was dramatically shifting the use of the facility. When the Parkview Center entrance was opened for outpatient services, the facility was faced with two "Main Entrances," one for inpatients and one for outpatients. A new wayfinding methodology was developed that used a quadrant system tied to the two entrances. The exterior signage substantially picked up architectural elements associated with each entrance: The "Main Entrance" had a sharp gable-roof detail, while the new "Parkview Entrance" sported a rounded architectural feature.

Exterior signs are designed with interchangeable panels even though they appear monolithic.

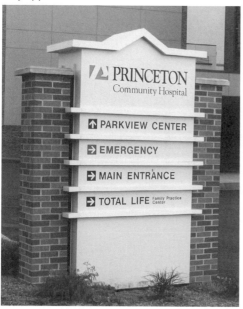

Exterior signs are internally illuminated with copy that appears black by day and white at night. The two main entrances have distinguishing shapes based on the entrance architecture, in this case an arched entry.

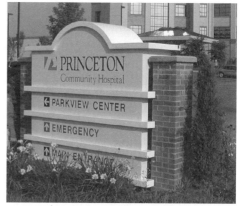

*Our thanks to Colleen Clark, director, Purchasing, Princeton Community Hospital, for providing this information.

Basics of wayfinding had not been emphasized. The introduction of a second set of public elevators and a second major entrance required a rethinking of how the facility was intended to function from a patient throughput perspective. As part of the wayfinding process, extensive staff interviews and training in conveying consistent, simple directions to visitors using common language were conducted.

Placemaking and interior accents were needed. Public signage incorporated solid-core accents to convey an upgraded aesthetic while not introducing a large cost factor, especially for

reorders, because frames stay in place while the ADA-compliant inserts are modular and easy to replace. Elevators were designated and identified to clearly indicate which bank of elevators transports visitors to which quadrant of the facility.

Exterior signage was outdated. The wayfinding team updated the old exterior signage with the corporate color scheme, unifying interior and exterior signage as well as displaying the facility logo for a more enhanced look. The new primary signage features interchangeable directional panels with type that appears black in the daytime and white (internally illuminated) at night.

Naming the primary elevator banks became a key to the success of the wayfinding program.

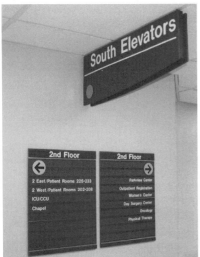

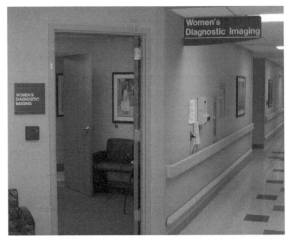

Overhead "blade" signs work hand in hand with smaller wall-mounted signs to identify major areas. Blade signs are visually clean and can be read from some distance.

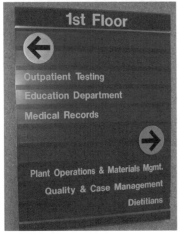

Directional modules feature easy-to-update insert strips with vinyl lettering.

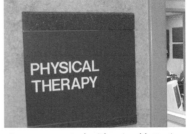

All room identification signs are created with raised lettering and Grade II Braille to guarantee ADA compliance. The insert can be removed without replacing the solid-core frame.

VALUE ENGINEERING: ROCKDALE MEDICAL CENTER, CONYERS, GEORGIA*

In 2003, Rockdale Medical Center (RMC) broke ground on its new East Tower, which would house multiple service lines and the main entrance of the facility, and changed its name from Rockdale Hospital and Health System to Rockdale Medical Center; a new logo also reflected the name change. The two events warranted new exterior signage, to guide patients and visitors to the correct entrance and the relocated services, and a new interior signage system for the new tower.

The RMC Signage Committee included the chief operating officer; the director of marketing and strategic planning; the director of facilities; the construction project manager; a representative of the architectural firm hired for the project; and the facility's communications coordinator, who served as project leader. The committee hired a well-respected architectural signage firm and set about to name the hospital's five entrances, three of them on the same side of the facility. Using a combination of compass points and service lines,

Visitor guides in English and Spanish provide floor plans to facilitate wayfinding while at the site.

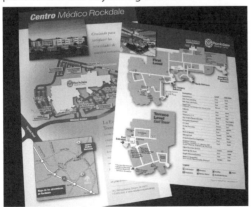

Photo courtesy of Med Maps, Inc.

> **At a Glance**
> Established: 1954
> Beds: 154
> Population served: 179,000
> Inpatient admissions: 8,268
> Outpatient visits: 111,441
> Employees: 738
> Square footage: 484,000

they settled on North, South, East (the main entrance), Emergency, and Day Surgery.

The marketing and physician relations departments undertook the responsibility to educate local physicians' staff on how to guide their patients to the correct location, using new directional maps that were distributed to the physician's offices and placed on the hospital's Web site.

The committee chose modular exterior signage to display the new entrance designations and an interior signage system that complemented the new tower's Planetree-inspired design. The result was aesthetically pleasing but, unfortunately, too expensive to use in the remainder of the facility as had been planned.

Once all the new construction was complete, RMC was faced with the dilemma of having five different interior signage systems, none of which was designed to allow for in-house maintenance. In 2006, RMC brought in a design consultant to perform a wayfinding needs survey and then develop an affordable sixth system that would complement the new one in the East Tower. The solution was card stock inserts that could be easily updated by RMC staff using existing software and laser printers, allowing changes to be made in minutes instead of weeks. This new system is being used for all new projects and to replace existing signage throughout the facility.

*Our thanks to Dave Stewart, former communications coordinator, Rockdale Medical Center (now employed by Cooper Signage & Graphics) for providing this information.

When a change in policy shifted the entrances used for labor and delivery patients and visitors, new exterior signage, using the value engineering recommendations, was installed to help reduce the confusion.

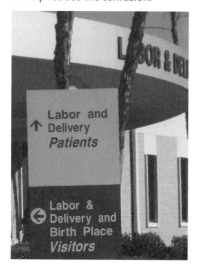

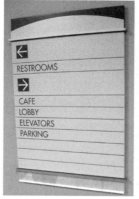
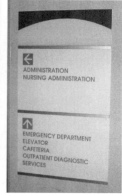

Image A   Image B

Tasked with expanding the newly implemented signage (as shown in image A) with a more flexible and more affordable program, the design consultant developed a generic version that was similar in appearance at much lower cost (as shown in image B) and that provided the capability to be updated in-house.

An integral part of the wayfinding program was to provide directional information on the facility's Web site to direct patients and visitors to the correct entrance.

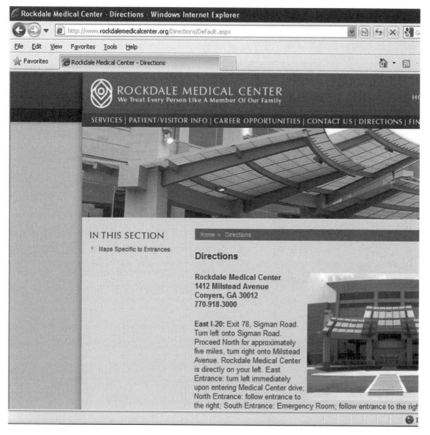

ADDRESS SYSTEM RESCUES LOST SIGNAGE PROGRAM: THE FINLEY HOSPITAL, IOWA HEALTH SYSTEM, DUBUQUE, IOWA*

The main campus of The Finley Hospital includes the hospital, Wendt Regional Cancer Center, and an MOB, all of which are interconnected.

Over the years, the hospital's signage system had been neglected. No one person was responsible for signage, each department and area was posting its own signage, and no numbering system was in place for rooms other than patient rooms. After five additions in the previous 50 years, finding one's way around the hospital was problematic; indeed, wayfinding was one of the top complaints on patient surveys.

Once approval was received to proceed with a wayfinding and signage study, a search was conducted and a consulting firm selected to perform the work. Its charge was to evaluate the current situation and develop recommendations for improving the wayfinding at Finley, including helping to create a room-numbering system for the hospital.

Following interviews with administration, managers, employees, patients, and visitors, the consultant recommended a wayfinding and numbering system based on a city street and address concept, as follows:

- Corridors were given the names of well-known streets in Dubuque.
- Departments were given a street address and numbers.
- Signage for departments and directional signs were put in place that resembled local street signs.

At a Glance
Established: 1890
Beds: 142
Population served: 90,000
Inpatient admissions: 8,610
Outpatient visits: 37,661
Employees: 930
Square footage: 247,335

- Department marker signs at entrances feature historical pictures of The Finley Hospital and its various departments.
- A scrolling digital electronic sign tells patients visiting the multi-use clinic on the third floor which type of clinic is being held that day. The sign is easily changed each day by clinic staff using a remote control device.

The lobby features a freestanding street sign directional module.

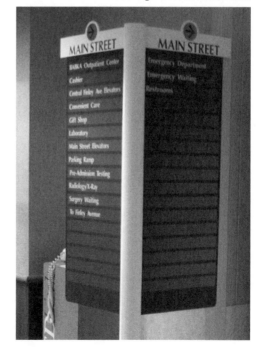

*Our thanks to Neal Erdmann, director, Facilities, The Finley Hospital, for providing this information.

Signposts were used to reinforce the hallways named for local roads in the directional program.

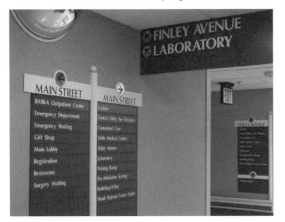

The results were immediate. The number of wayfinding complaints from patients and visitors has dropped virtually to zero. In fact, the hospital has received many compliments on the look and effectiveness of the new signs and directories. Identification of rooms and offices throughout the building has enhanced both life safety and energy management systems.

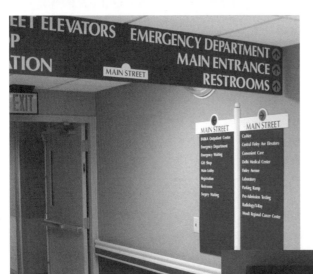

In the event that visitors do not pick up on the street numbering/naming concept, traditional left and right listings make wayfinding clear.

To make each major area unique, historic sepia-printed photos were used to add interest throughout the building.

PROJECTING HOPE THROUGH GENEROSITY: HOPE LODGES, AMERICAN CANCER SOCIETY, GEORGIA, NORTH CAROLINA, AND SOUTH CAROLINA*

More than most other hospital patients, cancer patients who have to travel to receive treatment often have a hard time finding a place to stay that can accommodate their special needs, let alone provide a home-like environment. The American Cancer Society's Hope Lodges do both, and do it for free, thanks to the generosity of donors who give time, money, and effort to make each lodge a reality.

How do you recognize that kind of generosity without making the structure feel like a mausoleum or museum? With the right kind of signage.

In addition to roomy suites with private baths, each Hope Lodge features shared kitchen and dining facilities, where patients and families can make their own meals and come together for support and comfort, as well as a game room, a business center, laundry facilities, a library, and quiet nooks. Signs bearing messages of dedication from donors identify these spaces, most of which have a personal name (e.g., The Sloan Reading Room).

In the reception area of most lodges, a "Friends Wall" honors donors in a fashion that fits with that location's unique decor. More than just a listing of names, the sign or signs

> At a Glance
> *Winn-Dixie Hope Lodge, Atlanta*
> Established: 1998
> Rooms: 52
> Square footage: 54,500
>
> *McConnell-Rabb Hope Lodge, Greenville, North Carolina*
> Established: 2002
> Rooms: 20
> Square footage: 28,000
>
> *Carol Grotnes Belk Campus Hope Lodge, Charleston, South Carolina*
> Established: 2002
> Rooms: 17
> Square footage: 14,000

allow guests to read a bit about the people who have made this home away from home possible. Each guest room bears the name of a donor as well, adding to the feeling of personalization.

The Hope Lodge wayfinding program starts with the American Cancer Society Web site, where browsers can take a virtual tour of any of the twenty-eight lodges. The Web address is http://www.cancer.org/docroot/subsite/hopelodge/index.asp.

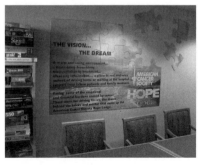

An environmental graphic decorates this "puzzle room" while conveying the lodge's mission statement.

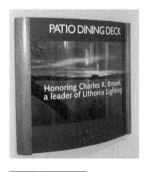

Every floor, area, and room identification plaque incorporates donor information. In one lodge, each sign features a unique photo picked by the donor and a unique verse or caption honoring the life of someone.

---

*Our thanks to Jim Donahue, president, R4 Resources for Facilities, Inc., for providing this information.

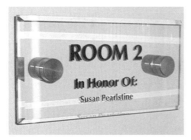

Hope Lodge in Charleston utilizes clear Plexiglas with standoffs at each door to honor donors.

In Atlanta, this environmental graphic emphasizes that while children are at the lodge, their swing set and other toys are anxiously awaiting their return to play.

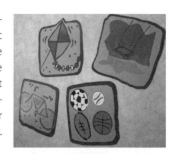

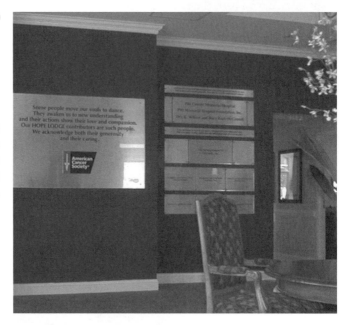

Brushed aluminum panels behind polished Plexiglas panels give strong emphasis to this hall of honor at the Greenville location.

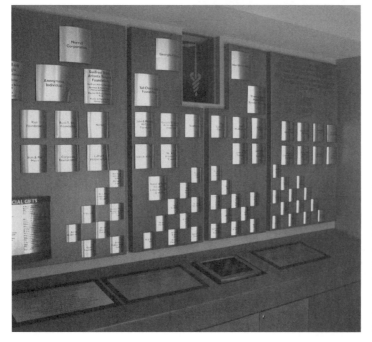

A donor hall of honor at the Atlanta location incorporates a touch screen unit to aid in direction finding in and around the lodge, as well as serving as a donor recognition tool. Other lodges have utilized clear Plexiglas or cast bronze plaques to honor their donors.

Sample Request for Wayfinding Consultation Proposal

I. **Information about firm**

Full corporate name _____

Address of headquarters _____

_____

_____

Phone number _____

Primary contact on this project _____

     Title _____

E-mail of primary contact _____

Firm Web site _____

Year established under this name _____

Primary services/products of firm _____

_____

_____

Type of business: Sole proprietorship, corporation (state in which incorporated _____), limited partnership, limited liability company, or other_____

Number of other locations you operate _____

Itemize total staff per location, and whether they are designer/management/support/ clerical/fabrication

List locations _____ , _____ , _____

Total billings for last year $ _____

Total billings last year for similar projects $_____ No. of facilities _____

Geographically, your primary service area is _____

II. **Staff information**

Attach brief biographies of key staff who will be directly involved in this project. Include experience, years with your firm, and area(s) of expertise.

III. Experience

(Health care ONLY, similar to this project in scope/size)

1. Facility _____ Size/number of beds _____

Location _____

Describe your scope of services, fees charged, and time frame in which accomplished.

_____

_____

_____

_____

Project coordinator for client _____ Phone _____

Discuss the client's problems and your approach to solving them.

_____

_____

_____

2. Facility _____ Size/number of beds _____

Location _____

Describe your scope of services, fees charged, and time frame in which accomplished.

_____

_____

_____

_____

Project coordinator for client _____ Phone _____

Discuss the client's problems and your approach to solving them.

_____

_____

_____

3. Facility _____ Size/number of beds _____

Location _____

Describe your scope of services, fees charged, and time frame in which accomplished.

_____

_____

_____

_____

Project coordinator for client _____ Phone _____

Discuss the client's problems and your approach to solving them.

_____

_____

_____

4. Facility _____ Size/number of beds _____

Location _____

Describe your scope of services, fees charged, and time frame in which accomplished.

_____

_____

_____

_____

Project coordinator for client _____ Phone _____

Discuss the client's problems and your approach to solving them.

_____

_____

_____

5. Facility _____ Size/number of beds _____

Location _____

Describe your scope of services, fees charged, and time frame in which accomplished.

_____

_____

_____

_____

Project coordinator for client _____ Phone _____

Discuss the client's problems and your approach to solving them.

_____

_____

_____

Number of health care wayfinding clients you had in the last year _____

The approximate combined dollar volume $ _____

Market segments in which you are involved:

☐ Acute care facilities   _____ % of your work

☐ Long-term care/nursing units   _____ % of your work

☐ Specialized medical facilities   _____ % of your work

☐ Hotels/motels   _____ % of your work

☐ Retail stores/gas stations   _____ % of your work

☐ Corporate/office complexes   _____ % of your work

☐ Airports/public facilities   _____ % of your work

☐ Real estate   _____ % of your work

☐ Museums/exhibits   _____ % of your work

☐ Churches/religious complexes   _____ % of your work

☐ Educational facilities   _____ % of your work

☐ Sales/service to the sign trade   _____ % of your work

☐ Other _____   _____ % of your work

☐ Other _____   _____ % of your work

Total should equal 100%

IV. Discuss your approach to our project, what opportunities you see as most formidable, and your plan to address them.

V. Current insurances/bonding

☐ Worker's compensation insurance, limits, and insurer name

_____

_____

☐ General liability insurance, limits, and insurer name

_____

_____

☐ Adequacy and accuracy insurance, limits, and insurer name

_____

_____

VI. Choose all services/products that you provide using your own staff:
*If your firm offers signage implementation services, you must complete a signage vendor qualification form and submit with this form.

- ☐ Provide wayfinding consultation
- ☐ Custom design based on client needs
- ☐ Program standard wayfinding elements
- ☐ Provide project management of wayfinding implementation
- ☐ *Fabricate signage _____ % interior _____ % exterior
- ☐ *Broker signage
- ☐ *Install signage
- ☐ Train client's staff as needed
- ☐ Equip and provide supplies as needed for in-house fabrication

State/federal/local licenses held

_____

_____

VII. List any lawsuits in which you are currently involved.

VIII. List any orders you canceled, projects from which you withdrew or on which you defaulted, or contracts you terminated within the past five years, and reason.

IX. List endorsements by health care organizations, group purchasing organizations, etc.

X. List recent awards and other peer recognition.

XI. List articles/books recently published and educational events recently produced/hosted.

XII. Discuss any factor that uniquely qualifies you for this project.

Typography 101

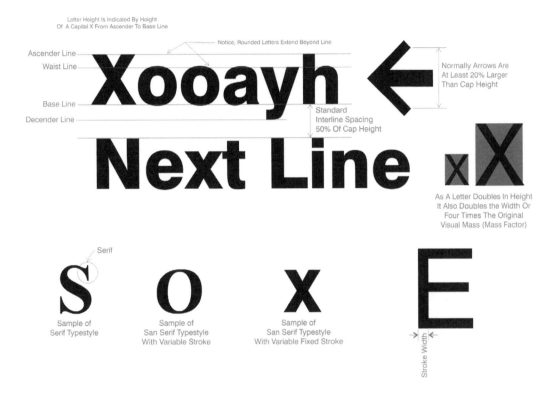

Letter Height Is Indicated By Height
Of A Capital X From Ascender To Base Line

Notice, Rounded Letters Extend Beyond Line

Ascender Line
Waist Line

Xooayh

Normally Arrows Are
At Least 20% Larger
Than Cap Height

Base Line
Decender Line

Standard
Interline Spacing
50% Of Cap Height

Next Line

As A Letter Doubles In Height
It Also Doubles the Width Or
Four Times The Original
Visual Mass (Mass Factor)

Serif

S O x E

Sample of
Serif Typestyle

Sample of
San Serif Typestyle
With Variable Stroke

Sample of
San Serif Typestyle
With Variable Fixed Stroke

Stroke Width

Initial Caps   Sentence case   ALL CAPS   lower case

Now is the time for
all good men to
come to the aid of
their country.

Flush Left Format

Now is the time for
all good men to
come to the aid of
their country.

Centered Format

Now is the time for
all good men to
come to the aid of
their country.

Flush Right Format

This is an example of 16 point type. Most consider this an adequate size for large print materials such as maps and printed directions. Notice the inter-character spacing is increased 10% for better readability.

ADA Typography

Examples Of Compliant ADA Fonts

ARIAL
AVANTE GARDE
SWISS 721
MICROSOFT SANS SERIF

Examples Of Non-compliant Fonts

ARIAL BLACK
CASLON
OPTIMA
TIMES ROMAN

Contrast & glare are critical to readibility
Contrast & glare are critical to readibility
Contrast & glare are critical to readibility
Contrast & glare are critical to readibility
Contrast & glare are critical to readibility

Signage Bidder Prequalification

This sample bidder prequalification questionnaire is meant not so much to elicit right or wrong answers as to gain knowledge of bidders' experience level.

The following are considerations in evaluating the responses received on the questionnaire:

- Did the bidder answer every question? If not, does it indicate the bidder has something to hide, or a poor approach to project management?
- Is the potential vendor large enough to handle your project? In a strong economy, a smaller company may be too busy with other projects. In a weak economy, it may downsize staff to the point at which it cannot serve you adequately.
- Does the bidder have extensive health care experience, similar in size and scope to your needs? You would not hire a contractor that builds houses to build a skyscraper, for example.
- What pieces does the company fabricate in-house, as the process relates to your needs? This question is most important when the project is nearing completion and changes to the signage are required. If the vendor has to order a new sign instead of going back to the shop and having it made quickly, your project could suffer lost time and incur additional cost.
- Is the organization stable? Will it be around to finish the project and be there when you have reorders?

Obviously, these are baseline questions, and you should customize them as needed. But a prequalification form is a powerful tool, and you will be glad you used it. It should be sent out to potential bidders at least two months ahead of final bid documents being issued so you have time to review and identify or disqualify potential bidders. Allow bidders about two weeks to respond.

SIGNAGE VENDOR PREQUALIFICATION FORM

I.   **Information about firm**

Full corporate name _____

Address of headquarters _____

_____

_____

Phone number _____

Primary contact on this project _____

        Title _____

E-mail of primary contact _____

Firm's Web site _____

Year established under this name _____

Primary services/products of your firm _____

_____

_____

Type of business: sole proprietorship, corporation (in what state incorporated _____),
limited partnership, limited liability company, or other_____

Is your business a franchisee?   □ Yes   □ No

If yes, where is franchisee headquartered? _____   How many units? _____

How many other locations do you own? _____

Itemize total staff per location and their function: designer/management/support/
clerical/fabrication

List locations _____ , _____ , _____
(Attach additional sheets if needed.)

Total billings for last year _____   Total health care billings last year _____

Total billings last year for similar projects _____   Number of facilities _____

Geographically, what is your primary service area? _____

Would you be willing to submit a current profit and loss statement?   □ Yes   □ No

II.   **Staff information**

Attach brief biographies of key staff who will be directly involved with this project.
Include experience, years with your firm, area(s) of expertise, and their role if selected
for this project.

III. Experience

(Health care ONLY, similar to this project in scope and size)

1. Facility _____ Size/number of beds _____

Location _____

Describe your scope of services, challenges faced, how you overcame challenges, fees charged, and time frame of completion:

_____

_____

_____

_____

Project coordinator for client _____ Phone _____

Discuss project's problems and your approach to solving them:

_____

_____

_____

2. Facility _____ Size/number of beds _____

Location _____

Describe your scope of services, challenges faced, how you overcame challenges, fees charged, and time frame of completion:

_____

_____

_____

_____

Project coordinator for client _____ Phone _____

Discuss project's problems and your approach to solving them:

_____

_____

_____

3. Facility _____ Size/number of beds _____

Location _____

Describe your scope of services, challenges faced, how you overcame challenges, fees charged, and time frame of completion:

_____

_____

_____

_____

Project coordinator for client _____ Phone _____

Discuss project's problems and your approach to solving them:

_____

_____

_____

4. Facility _____ Size/number of beds _____

Location _____

Describe your scope of services, challenges faced, how you overcame challenges, fees charged, and time frame of completion:

_____

_____

_____

_____

Project coordinator for client _____ Phone _____

Discuss project's problems and your approach to solving them:

_____

_____

_____

5. Facility _____ Size/number of beds _____

Location _____

Describe your scope of services, challenges faced, how you overcame challenges, fees charged, and time frame of completion:

_____

_____

_____

_____

Project coordinator for client _____ Phone _____

Discuss project's problems and your approach to solving them:

_____

_____

_____

How many health care wayfinding clients did you have in the last year? _____

What is the approximate combined dollar volume (last year only) _____

Market segments in which you are involved:

☐ Acute health care facilities   _____ % of your work

☐ Long-term care/nursing units   _____ % of your work

☐ Specialized medical facilities   _____ % of your work

☐ Hospitality (hotels/motels)   _____ % of your work

☐ Retail stores/gas stations   _____ % of your work

☐ Corporate/office complexes   _____ % of your work

☐ Airports/public facilities   _____ % of your work

☐ Real estate   _____ % of your work

☐ Museums/exhibits   _____ % of your work

☐ Churches/religious complexes   _____ % of your work

☐ Educational facilities   _____ % of your work

☐ Sales/service to the sign trade   _____ % of your work

☐ Other _____   _____ % of your work

☐ Other _____   _____ % of your work

Total should equal 100%

IV. Discuss your approach to our project.
What opportunities do you see as most formidable? (Attach additional sheet if needed.)

V. Discuss your approach to change orders and cost containment.

VI. Current insurances/bonding:

☐ Worker's compensation insurance limits and insurance carrier:

_____

_____

☐ General liability insurance limits and insurance carrier:

_____

_____

☐ Adequacy and accuracy insurance limits and insurance carrier:

_____

_____

☐ Bid/performance bonding limits and available amount:

_____

_____

☐ Other (itemize)

_____

_____

VII. Signage fabrication

What percentage of your products are _____ % interior _____ % exterior?

What percentage of signage do you routinely fabricate in-house? _____

Interior signage products/process

_____ % Photopolymer Americans with Disabilities Act (ADA)–compliant plaques

_____ % Raster ADA-compliant plaques

_____ % Directional modules

_____ % Illuminated directories

_____ % Non-illuminated directories

_____ % Touch screen directories/kiosks

_____ % High-definition signage

_____ % Engraving

_____ % Silkscreening

_____ % Hotstamping

_____ % Digital prints

_____ % Vinyl

_____ % Photo/acid etch

_____ % Injection molded

_____ % Custom fabrication

_____ % Other—please indicate: _____

_____

Exterior signage products/process

_____ % Post and panel modules

_____ % Aluminum extrusions for cabinets

_____ % Sheet metal cabinetry

_____ % Channel letters/logos:

      Do you produce neon lettering in-house?   ☐ Yes   ☐ No

      Do you produce LED (light-emitting diode) signage in-house?
      ☐ Yes   ☐ No

_____ % Flat-cut letters/logos

_____ % Fiberglass monoliths

_____ % Architectural foam/stucco monoliths

_____ % Electronic message centers

_____ % Production fabrication

_____ % Custom fabrication

_____ % Wood signage

_____ % Other—please indicate: _____

_____

Please list major equipment you have in-house:

_____

_____

_____

Do you manufacture UL (Underwriters Laboratories)–labeled products?
☐ Yes, in-house   ☐ No   ☐ Not in-house, but available

What types of signage do you not fabricate and broker?

_____

_____

_____

_____

Services

☐ Install signage with your own crews.
  List equipment:_____

☐ Train client's staff as needed.

☐ Equip and provide supplies as needed for in-house fabrication.

State/federal/local licenses held:

_____

_____

VIII. Are you currently involved in any lawsuits? Explain.

_____

 IX. List any canceled orders, any projects from which you withdrew, or any projects
      or contracts on which you defaulted within the past five years. Explain.

_____

_____

_____

_____

  X. List group purchasing organizations with which you are currently under contract:

 XI. List endorsements by health care organizations:

XII. List recent awards and other peer recognition:

XIII. List articles/books recently published by or about you and other educational
       events hosted:

XIV. Discuss any experience that uniquely qualifies you for this project.

Would you be willing to sign a noncollusion agreement with anyone involved with the design
team, project management team, and facility?   ☐ Yes   ☐ No

ADA Basics
Related to Signage*

The new ADA Accessibility Guidelines [ADAAG] are significantly more stringent in the area of typography for the blind. Reading tactile letters is extremely difficult. The letters must be relatively consistent in size and shape on every sign in the environment in order to be easily read. Tactile letters must also be smaller in size and simpler than most visual letters in the environment.

Tactile type, though, applies only to permanent room identification signs; these apply to rooms that will not change names for at least a year.

HEIGHT OF TACTILE LETTERS

There is only a narrow band of allowable heights for tactile letters: 5/8″ minimum and 2″ maximum based on the letter "I" (703.2.5). Tactile letters must always be capitalized.

Tactile letters must also be minimum 1/32″ in height from the surface of the sign. They may be beveled or chamfered.

CHARACTER PROPORTION AND STROKE WIDTH

Tactile letters must be san serif and always capitalized. Characters must be selected from fonts where the width of the uppercase letter "O" is 55 percent minimum and 110 percent maximum of the height of the uppercase letter "I" at the top of the tactile text (703.5.4). The stroke width may be only 15% maximum of the height of the letter "I" (703.5.6). This rule makes most san serif fonts not permissible for use, including Times Roman, bold font, and Optima. Stroke width rules are only for the top of tactile letters. If bold characters are beveled, they may comply.

Under the new ADAAG, very few fonts are allowed. Test each font's stroke width to be sure.

LETTER SPACING

Character spacing is measured between the two closest points of adjacent tactile characters within a message, excluding word spaces. For unbeveled letters, there must be a 1/8″ minimum spacing between letters and a maximum spacing of 4 times the letter stroke width. When characters are beveled, there must be a 1/16″ spacing

*Excerpted from "ADA White Paper Update: 2006 Guidelines, Best Practices, and Innovation for Signs for the Blind and Visually Impaired." Reprinted with permission of the Society for Environmental Graphic Design (SEGD).

minimum at the letter base with 4 times the stroke width maximum at the base (703.2.7).

Spacing requirements for the top of the letters are the same as for unbeveled letters. Characters must be separated from raise borders and decorative elements by 3/8 inch minimum. . . .

WHEN TO USE TACTILE FONTS EXCLUSIVELY

Tactile type fonts and visual fonts can be the same, but it is important to determine in which environments they work the best in combination. Buildings with narrow hallways and repetitive room numbers have little need for identification signs that can be seen from a great distance. Buildings like hotels, office buildings, and residential structures may fit these criteria. Buildings that have large open spaces to be navigated, have unique destination names, or contain extensive temporary information may need to split tactile signs [from] visual signs.

The ADAAG rules defining typography for the sighted are much less restrictive than those for the blind, but they are required on a greater variety of signs, including permanent and temporary identification, directory, and directional signs. Any type font is permissible for visual signs, using both capital and lower case letters, as long as they do not conflict with the guidelines for tactile type.

MINIMUM LETTER HEIGHTS

The most current ADAAG defines letter heights in far more detail than previous versions, focusing on the height of letters in a variety of sign heights and distances. The most important element when designing using these heights is minimum ground clearance. Most wall mounted directional signs need only use the 5/8″ minimum letter heights, while most ceiling mounted directional signs must use letter heights of 2″ or more. . . .

MULTI-LINGUAL AND SYMBOL LETTER HEIGHTS

There are currently no requirements for letter heights on multi-lingual signs. It is advisable when using multiple languages to have them all include legible letter heights. For symbols, the use of a dominant symbol still requires following legible letter height rules. And smaller type permissible on symbol signs may still be permissible under the current ADAAG, depending on how the state and local codes interpret the guidelines. . . .

DUAL SIGNS

For the first time, ADAAG has recognized that signs for the blind and the visually impaired require two different types of sign: small san serif tactile letters for the blind and larger letters with greater color contrast for the visually impaired. These two distinct needs are encapsulated in recommendation 703.1, which clarifies that both visual and tactile letters of different heights can be placed on the same sign. This frees the designer from being restricted to a very narrow window for type heights and styles. When designing a dual sign, it is important to remember that tactile letters and Braille must be between 48″ from the Braille base and 60″ from the top of the tactile letter off the floor (703.4.1), although the visual text can be anywhere on the sign. On the other hand, visual text must have a color contrast with its background of at least 60%, while no color contrast is needed at all for tactile signs. Visual signs are open to any type font, but the restrictions on tactile letters remain. One easing of the rules on tactile type is allowing dual signs to use tactile letter heights as opposed to the 5/8″ minimum employed on signs where visual and tactile text are the same. Because of the distinct needs of visual versus tactile signs, it is important to have a strategy when employing these signs. Even [though] additional information (including temporary room information) can be placed on a dual sign, it is important that permanent room identification be consistent between visual and tactile elements. . . .

[SEGD] RECOMMENDATIONS:

- Depending on the environment, it may be important to create different typography for both the blind and the visually impaired. Transportation facilities and convention centers need distinct type for each group; in hotels and repetitive offices it is impossible to combine them.
- The top of tactile fonts is what the blind read and where stroke width and spacing rules must be met.
- Only a narrow set of typefaces are allowed for tactile signs. All typefaces are allowed for visual signs as long as they are the right height.
- Visual typography rules apply to all sign types, including overhead signs that must be read from a distance.
- Typography for the blind must be capitalized. It is recommended (but not required) to use upper and lower case when designing visible type faces. Here are excerpts we should use from section five (same white paper):

Color Contrast

The ADAAG recommends a 70% Light Reflectance Value (LRV) (Appendix to Part 1192), but this is not a strict requirement.

There are a number of color combinations in the 60–70% range that work well, which is why 70% is not a requirement.

The Position of Braille and Tactile Text on Signs

Braille is positioned directly below the lowest tactile text, in one line if possible (703.3.2). Braille must be no less than 48″ off the floor (703.4.1). Since the baseline of tactile must be no more than 60″ off the floor, this permits only a small window for both text and Braille. When tactile text is on multiple lines, the Braille should be on one line, 3/8″ below the bottom line of the text. (Only one line of tactile text is strongly suggested for permanent room identification.) For elevator buttons, Braille need only be located as close to the 60″ mark as possible to meet the needs of most adult users. Facilities geared to children (such as schools and children's hospitals) should locate text closer to the 48″ height.

Use of Sequential Numbers and Letters

Because tactile readers take so long to read a sign, and because numbers can be understood sequentially, it is encouraged that room numbers and letters should be used for room recognition purposes, with any other descriptions used as supplementary material. If tactile text is being used with supplementary visual text on the same sign, it is important that Braille be placed in close proximity to tactile text, even though the ADAAG does not define a maximum distance between Braille and tactile letters.

Position of Tactile Text on Signs

Tactile text is strictly regulated by the ADAAG. All tactile text must be positioned with the bottom of the tactile letter at least 3/8″ above the Braille, and the baseline of the tactile letter no more than 60″ off the floor (703.4.1). Text must be at least 3/8″ away from the closest raised border or rule line. (These rules do not apply to elevator controls.) For multiple lines of text, letter spacing from the top line must be no less than 35% and no more than 70% of the text height. (The specific text mandates a spacing of 135% to 170% of text height from baseline to baseline of multi-line text [703.2.8].) For example, 1″ letters on multiple lines should be no less than about 1/3″ and no more than about 2/3″ apart.

No Vertical Tactile Text!

Although it is not expressly prohibited in the ADAAG, vertical tactile text and numbers should not be used.

Position of Tactile Signs

Since all identification of permanent rooms and spaces is required to be tactile, the ADAAG provides specific instructions on the location of tactile signs for room doors and entrances (703.4.2).

EXCERPTS FROM ADA-ABA ACCESSIBILITY GUIDELINES

[For more information, visit http://www.access-board.gov/ada-aba/final.cfm.]

703 Signs

703.1 General. Signs shall comply with 703. Where both visual and tactile characters are required, either one sign with both visual and tactile characters, or two separate signs, one with visual, and one with tactile characters, shall be provided.

703.2 Raised Characters. Raised characters shall comply with 703.2 and shall be duplicated in Braille complying with 703.3. Raised characters shall be installed in accordance with 703.4.

Advisory: 703.2 Raised Characters. Signs that are designed to be read by touch should not have sharp or abrasive edges.

703.2.1 Depth. Raised characters shall be 1/32 inch (0.8mm) minimum above their background.

703.2.2 Case. Characters shall be uppercase.

703.2.3 Style. Characters shall be sans serif. Characters shall not be italic, oblique, script, highly decorative, or of other unusual forms.

703.2.4 Character Proportions. Characters shall be selected from fonts where the width of the uppercase letter "O" is 55 percent minimum and 2 inches (51mm) maximum based on the height of the uppercase letter "I".

Figure 703.2.5. Height of Raised Characters

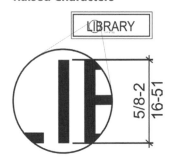

703.2.5 Character Height. Character height measured vertically from the baseline of the character shall be 5/8 inch (16mm) minimum and 2 inches (51mm) maximum based on the height of the uppercase letter "I".

EXCEPTION: Where separate raised and visual characters with the same information are provided, raised character height shall be permitted to be ½ inch (13mm) minimum.

703.2.6 Stroke Thickness. Stroke thickness of the uppercase letter "I" shall be 15 percent maximum of the height of the character.

703.2.7 Character Spacing. Character spacing shall be measured between the two closest points of adjacent raised characters within a message, excluding word spaces. Where characters have rectangular cross sections, spacing between individual raised characters shall be 1/8 inch (3.2 mm) minimum and 4 times the raised character stroke width maximum. Where characters have other cross sections, spacing between individual raised characters shall be 1/16 inch (1.6mm) minimum and 4 times the raised character stroke width maximum at the base of the cross sections, and 1/8 inch (3.2 mm) minimum and 4 times the raised character stroke width maximum at the top of the cross sections. Characters shall be separated from raised borders and decorative elements 3/8 inch (9.5mm) minimum.

703.2.8 Line Spacing. Spacing between the baselines of separate lines of raised characters within a message shall be 135 percent minimum and 170 percent maximum of the raised character height.

703.3 Braille. Braille shall be contracted (Grade 2) [and] shall comply with 703.3 and 703.4.

703.3.1 Dimensions and Capitalization. Braille dots shall have a domed or rounded shape and shall comply with Table 703.3.1. The indication of an uppercase letter or letters shall only be used before the first word of sentences, proper nouns and names, individual letters of the alphabet, initials, and acronyms.

703.3.1. Braille Dimensions

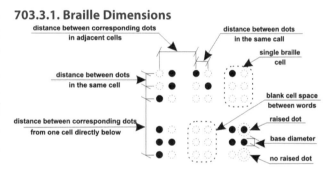

Figure 703.3.1. Braille Measurement

Measurement Range *(Measured center to center)*	Minimum, in Inches
Dot base diameter	0.059 (1.5mm) to …
Distance between two dots in the same cell	0.090 (2.3mm) to 0.100 (2.5mm)
Distance between corresponding dots	0.241 (6.1mm) to 0.300 (7.6mm)
Dot height	0.025 (0.6mm) to …
Distance between corresponding dots from one cell directly below	0.395 (10mm) to 0.400 (10.2mm)

Figure 703.3.2. Position of Braille

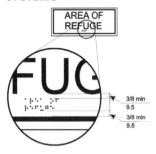

703.3.2 Position. Braille shall be positioned below the corresponding text. If text is multi-lined, Braille shall be placed below the entire text. Braille shall be separated 3/8 inch (9.5mm) minimum from any other tactile characters and 3/8 inch (9.5mm) minimum from raised borders and decorative elements.

EXCEPTION: Braille provided on elevator [car] controls shall be separated 3/16 inch (4.8mm) minimum and shall be located either directly below or adjacent to the corresponding raised characters or symbols.

703.4 Installation Height and Location. Signs with tactile characters shall comply with 703.4.

703.4.1 Height above Finish Floor or Ground. Tactile characters on signs shall be located 48 inches (1220mm) minimum above the finish floor or ground surface, measured from the baseline of the lowest tactile character and 60 inches (1525mm) maximum above the finish floor or ground surface, measured from the baseline of the highest tactile character.

Figure 703.4.1. Height of Tactile Characters above Finish Floor or Ground

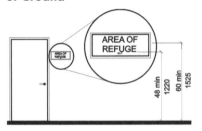

EXCEPTION: Tactile characters for elevator car controls shall not be required to comply with 703.4.1.

703.4.2 Location. Where a tactile sign is provided at a door, the sign shall be located alongside the door at the latch side. Where a tactile sign is provided at double doors with one active leaf, the sign shall be located on the inactive leaf. Where a tactile sign is provided at double doors with two active leafs, the sign shall be located to the right of the right hand door. Where there is no wall space at the latch side of a single door or at the right side of double doors, signs shall be located on the nearest adjacent wall. Signs containing tactile characters shall be located so that a clear floor space of 18 inches (455mm) minimum by 18 inches (455mm) minimum, centered on the tactile characters, is provided beyond the arc of any door swing between the closed position and 45 degree open position.

Figure 703.4.2. Location of Tactile Signs at Doors

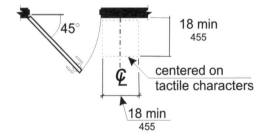

EXCEPTION: Signs with tactile characters shall be permitted on the push side of doors with closers and without hold-open devices.

703.5 Visual Characters. Visual characters shall comply with 703.5.

EXCEPTION: Where visual characters comply with 703.2 and are accompanied by Braille complying with 703.3, they shall not be required to comply with 703.5.2 through 703.5.9.

703.5.1 Finish and Contrast. Characters and their background shall have a non-glare finish. Characters shall contrast with their background with either light characters on a dark background or dark characters on a light background.

Advisory: 703.5.1 Finish and Contrast. Signs are more legible for persons with low vision when characters contrast as much as possible with their background. Additional factors affecting the ease with which the text can be distinguished from its background include shadows cast by lighting sources, surface glare, and the uniformity of the text and its background colors and textures.

703.5.2 Case. Characters shall be uppercase or lowercase or a combination of both.

703.5.3 Style. Characters shall be conventional in form. Characters shall not be italic, oblique, script, highly decorative, or of other unusual forms.

703.5.4 Character Proportions. Characters shall be selected from fonts where the width of the uppercase letter "O" is 55 percent minimum and 110 percent maximum of the height of the uppercase letter "I".

703.5.5 Character Height. Minimum character height shall comply with Table 703.5.5. Viewing distance shall be measured as the horizontal distance between the character and an obstruction preventing further approach towards the sign. Character height shall be based on the uppercase letter "I".

703.5.6 Height from Finish Floor or Ground. Visual characters shall be 40 inches (1015mm) minimum above the finish floor or ground.

EXCEPTION: Visual characters indicating elevator car controls shall not be required to comply with 703.5.6.

703.5.7 Stroke Thickness. Stroke thickness of the uppercase letter "I" shall be 10 percent minimum and 30 percent maximum of the height of the character.

703.5.8 Character Spacing. Character spacing shall be measured between the two closest points of adjacent characters, excluding word spaces. Spacing between individual characters shall be 10 percent minimum and 35 percent maximum of character height.

703.5.9 Line Spacing. Spacing between the baselines of separate lines of characters within a message shall be 135 percent minimum and 170 percent maximum of the character height.

703.6 Pictograms. Pictograms shall comply with 703.6.

703.6.1 Pictogram Field. Pictograms shall have a field height of 6 inches (150mm) minimum. Characters and Braille shall not be located in the pictogram field.

703.6.2 Finish and Contrast. Pictograms and their field shall have a non-glare finish. Pictograms shall contrast with their field with either a light pictogram on a dark field or a dark pictogram on a light field.

Advisory: 703.6.2 Finish and Contrast. Signs are more legible for persons with low vision when characters contrast as much as possible with their background. Additional factors affecting the ease with which the text can be distinguished from its background include shadows cast by lighting sources, surface glare, and the uniformity of the text and background colors and textures.

703.6.3 Text Descriptors. Pictograms shall have text descriptors located directly below the pictogram field. Text descriptors shall comply with 703.2, 703.3, and 703.4.

703.7 Symbols of Accessibility. Symbols of accessibility shall comply with 703.7.

703.7.2 Symbols.

Figure 703.6.1. Pictogram Field

Volume Control Telephone

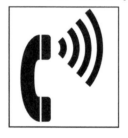

International Symbol of Access for Hearing Loss

International Symbol of Text Telephone (TTY)

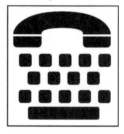

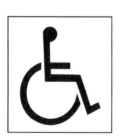

International Symbol of Accessibility

Spanish Translations of Commonly Used English Text

Please note: Translations are provided in good faith. However, all translations should be verified by your in-house language experts prior to implementation.

SHORTER TEXT

Ambulance Entrance	*Ingreso de Ambulancias*
Billing Department	*Departamento de Facturación*
Cardiology	*Cardiología*
Care Staff Area	*Área del Personal de Cuidado*
Center for Rehabilitative Medicine	*Centro de Medicina Rehabilitativa*
Chapel	*Capilla*
Conference Room	*Sala de Conferencias*
DECONTAMINATION	*DESCONTAMINACIÓN*
Diabetes (Education)	*Diabetes (Educación)*
Emergency	*Emergencia*
Emergency Center	*Centro de Emergencias*
Environmental Services	*Servicios Ambientales*
Extended Recovery	*Recuperación Prolongada*
Family Practice Clinic	*Clínica de Practica Familiar*
Family Room	*Cuarto de Familia*
Immunizations	*Immunizaciones*
Infectious Disease	*Enfermedades Infecciosas*
Intensive Care	*Cuidado Intensivo*
Internal Medicine	*Medicina Interna*
Interpretive Services	*Servicios Interpretacion*
Laboratory	*Laboratorio*
Main Entrance	*Entrada Principal*
Mammography	*Mamografía*

Medical Records	*Archivos Médicos*
Neurodiagnostic Lab	*Laboratorio de Neurodiagnóstico*
Patient Check-Out	*Salida del Paciente*
Patient Exit	*Salida de Pacientes*
Physicians Only	*Médicos Solamente*
Radiology/X-ray	*Radiologia/Rayos X*
Satellite Pharmacy	*Farmacia Satélite*
Short Stay	*Estancia Corta*
Staff Only	*Solamente Personal*
Surgery Waiting	*Área de Espera de Cirugiá*

LONGER TEXT

For Handicap Assistance, Please Push Button Below

Asistencia para personas incapacitadas, por favor presione el botón de abajo

FOR YOUR SAFETY:

If you are the patient, please ask the triage nurse before eating or drinking anything.

Por tu seguridad:

Si eres el paciente, por favor preguntale a la Enfermera de Triage antes de comer o tomar algo.

Limit 2 Visitors per Patient

Limite 2 visitantes por paciente

If you have a medical emergency or are in labor, even if you cannot pay or do not have medical insurance or you are not entitled to Medicare or Medicaid, you have the right to receive, within the capabilities of this hospital's staff and facilities:

- An appropriate medical screening examination;
- Necessary stabilization treatment (including treatment for an unborn child); and, if necessary,
- An appropriate transfer to another facility.

This hospital does participate in the Medicaid program.

Si usted tiene una emergencia medica o si esta en trabajo de parto, aun si usted no puede pagar ni tiene seguro medico y no califica para Medicare o Medicaid, usted tiene el derecho de recibir, dentro de las capacidades del personal de este hospital, lo siguiente:

- *Una evaluacion medica adecuada*
- *Tratamiento necesario para estabilizacion (incluyendo tratamientos para ninos aun no nacidos), y si se requiere*
- *Transferencia adecuada a otra institucion*

Este hospital participa en el Programa Medicaid.

Glossary

Every industry has jargon or a unique usage of words. Although this glossary is nothing close to exhaustive, it provides a list of terms and phrases that will help you navigate the world of an environmental graphic designer.

ADA Americans with Disabilities Act

Bid documents Documents prepared for the express purpose of obtaining competitive bids and to act as legal documentation against which to measure a vendor's performance. These usually include specifications that detail performance criteria, message schedules (see *message schedule* below), location prints, and sign type drawings.

Camera-ready art/electronic art Artwork that is prepared in a format compatible with sign-making machines. This usually means type converted to curves (paths) and not in .jpg or bitmap format.

Channel letters The most prevalent use of channel letters is in retail/mall lettering. A letterform is backlighted in neon or light-emitting diodes (LEDs). These may have remote-located transformers or can be mounted onto a raceway (linear box) to contain the electrical components.

Control drawings Also called design intent drawings, these show the size, basic appearance/format, and other characteristics that communicate the designer's vision of the end product. These are not to be confused with bid documents.

Creative rights Most designers are sensitive to what information can be shared, especially for the use of competitive bidding. Simply stated, if you do not reach clear agreement with the designer that you will share intellectual materials (designs, etc.), then you may not legally or morally do so. Most documents are protected under U.S. copyright laws. (Please check before you reproduce/circulate documents.)

Decision point Along a pathway, this is an intersection, or an extended straight stretch, where one asks the question, "What do I do now, turn or continue to go straight?"

Directory versus directionals *Directories* primarily indicate vertical information, such as floor and suite location. *Directionals* orient the viewer on one horizontal plane, giving directions to go right, left, straight, and so forth.

Disbursements The tangible items supplied as a result of design consultation, such as a sign systems manual, electronic disks, hard copies, and so forth.

Electrical at site Most codes require that electric work performed at site, including trenching and cabling to the sign, be performed by a licensed electrician. Some codes allow the sign installer to connect the sign if it is within a few feet of the power source.

Environmental graphic design The discipline of planning, designing, and executing graphic elements in the natural and built spaces. This includes signage, displays, and related communicative tools.

Grade II Braille While Grade I Braille does not use contractions and abbreviations, Grade II does.

Illuminated/Non-illuminated Illumination is achieved in several ways:

> *Internally illuminated/backlighted* A portion of the sign/letter face is translucent, allowing lights in the sign structure to shine through the face. Common lighting options include high-output fluorescent bulbs, sodium vapor, neon, or LED, depending on the application.

> *Floodlighted* A non-illuminated sign can have floodlights washing the sign face and structure.

> *Ambient lighting* Depending on the ambient light available, hours of operation, and other conditions, some signs will not require any supplemental illumination. An application to consider is reflective letters/background to allow for headlights to bring the sign to life.

> *Silhouette illuminated* Most common with individual letters/logos, this method uses an opaque letter with concealed lighting behind it to create a halo effect.

> *Edge lighted* Acrylic will illuminate some signage based on internal refraction, mainly of etched or engraved images, to project a glow around the graphics.

Interactive signs Kiosks or other devices that allow two-way interaction in seeking information in wayfinding.

LED Light-emitting diode, an alternate light source being used in sign lighting, primarily to achieve low electrical consumption and ease of maintenance.

Lexicon The montage of the various sign types used in a given sign system. A lexicon is often an illustration that shows the interrelation of the elements used.

Line of sight Viewing from specific decision points to potential sign locations to determine the best possible signage placement.

Message schedule The document that lists the specific text for each sign that corresponds to a specific location on a location print.

Modular components Standard sign modules that feature interchangeable elements, most typically insert plaques or exterior systems of extruded aluminum (e.g., post and panel systems). Often the modules are designed to stack or sit side by side to appear as a preplanned grouping.

Monolith Usually refers to an exterior sign constructed in such a way as to appear to be one seamless piece. A semi-monolith is similar, with some seams or exposed fasteners.

Permit/over-the-counter permit A document issued by the appropriate agency allowing a sign to be built and erected in a specific location based on guidelines that regulate quantities, size placement, and other factors. Most codes allow for an appeal process known as a variance if the sign(s) is not compliant but is needed. This is often a complicated, expensive process and has no guarantee of success.

Post and panel units Exterior modular signs composed of aluminum extrusion sign posts, cabinets, and sign faces/panels.

Preferred path Not necessarily the shortest pathway from point A to point B. Instead, it is the path chosen for the purposes of giving directions. These paths should be visitor-friendly and create as positive an impression as possible along the way.

Programming versus design *Programming* signs is most often associated with taking standard catalog items and plugging them into places where they will be effective as communicative tools. *Design* is associated with the process of creating unique signage elements to address specific parameters.

Raceway The "box" on which internally illuminated letters are mounted to provide a place to run wires and other electrical components. Raceways may be visible or mounted as remote or concealed structures.

Retainer An L-shaped lip, mounted to the edge of a non-monolithic sign cabinet, that usually is removable to allow a sign face to slide in and out of a sign cabinet (or can) for ease of updating and service. Sometimes an access panel is used instead of a retainer (most often in monoliths) to allow access to electrical components.

Setback The distance that a sign or development code requires a sign to be placed behind a right-of-way or property line. This is measured in a straight line from the line to the part of the sign closest to the line.

Shop drawings Drawings prepared by sign vendors to detail exactly how they propose to construct and install signs. Once shop drawings are submitted, the client has three courses of action: to (1) approve, (2) approve as noted, or (3) revise and resubmit per notes provided. These are project specific and should not be confused with typical details.

Streetscape Collectively, all visual elements related to the curb appeal, including signs, traffic lights, mailboxes, bus stops, architectural features, trash receptacles, and landscaping.

Subsurface Application of lettering or images to the back or second surface of clear or frosted clear materials, such as plastic or glass. Often the background is painted to provide a contrast for the image and to provide an opaque background, which can allow for concealment of double-faced tape mounting.

Tactile lettering A term used by accessibility codes such as ADA to describe 1/32"-thick letterforms that can be traced with a finger to be readable to the blind or those of low vision.

Variance See *permit*.

Vertical paths Stairs, elevators, and escalators to move people from one horizontal plane to another (floor to floor).

Window signs 1. Interior plaques that utilize double-faced tape or other materials to create a gap that allows an insert to slide in and out easily for quick updating. The window acts as a picture frame that displays the insert plaque. 2. Signs displayed in a window, such as OPEN/CLOSED.

Index

Page numbers in italic refer to illustrations.